Fitness and Health

Boost gut health and immunity with a delicious approach to wellness that nourishes your mind, body and spirit.

Melanie Rivera

Contents............................**Errore. Il segnalibro non è definito.**

Today's Concerns about Wellness and Fitness

In this wonderful age of enlightenment and advanced medicines, we should be some of the most fit, most well human beings. But, you will most often find the opposite is true. So how and why has this happened? The following report takes a look at all the components that must be present for us to be fit and well. We will examine all the necessary conditions that must be met in order for us to be fit and well. And some of the more creative, fun and unique forms that self-help and medicine have taken over the last several centuries.

As you read the following paragraphs, we're going to walk through some of the more generalized areas of wellness, fitness and overall good health that each and every person should strive to attain. We'll then move on to examining the various areas of individual concern, fitness, wellness, the mind, body and soul importance, and the development of good health practices. All of these areas are necessary for the whole wellness of the individual.

The Blissful Union of Wellness and Fitness

You pick up the magazines each day, and you're bombarded with health and fitness information. Advertisements and articles that are designed to impart much needed information to the reader about the state of fitness and health in America today, and what we as responsible citizens should do. I want you to stop, and think for just one moment. How do you determine your current fitness and wellness levels? Does your regular doctor impart this information as you visit, does he inquire each time you go if you believe yourself to be fit and well? Probably not. Nor does he give you any method for determining the status on your own. Fitness centers abound in this country, and most are staffed with counselors who can test your fitness level. What about your wellness level? Are they one and the same? They are not one and the same, yet they rely heavily on each other to keep you healthy.

Thanks to the advances in modern medicine, the average person's life span now exceeds seventy years. If you stop to think, that's quite a long time to walk around on this earth. Along with the wonderful life expectancy increases, however have come the detrimental effects of overeating and unhealthy eating. It seems that as we advance in one area, we regress in others. This doesn't have to be so, however. Reaching a place of responsibility, where we combine our physical health, with our wellness enhances those extra years of life.

Being fit and being well are totally different conditions. Your wellness rating is dependent upon your immune system, and what vitamins, supplements, and nutrition you provide for your immune system. Fit people can sometimes be unwell. And well people can sometimes be unfit. However, when you do combine the two, and use sound principles based on clean living, exercise, and healthy eating, you attain a state of equilibrium where you are both fit and well. It is comparable to the Chinese philosophy of yin and yang. The balance that must exist in the whole relies heavily on the balancing of the halves.

The wonderful state that is attained however, when we are both fit and well, is one of the joys of being alive. The energy levels that we experience are beyond compare, and the happiness we feel during our moments of physical triumphs, help us to put life in perspective. That's an accomplishment we pass along to our children in the example that we set before them. We are true practitioners of the philosophies that we preach.

The example we provide for our family, our children especially, speaks volumes to them about their own responsibilities in maintaining their health. Being healthy is a true combination of wellness and fitness, body and mind. Our spirit, soul, or inner voice is a benefactor in this experience, also. Truly well and fit minds and bodies are better followers of their spirit, and spend more energy on the wellness of their spiritual aspect, also. Spirituality is a way of assuring ourselves of a renewing, and rebirth of ourselves as caring humans. Wellness encompasses our state of being, mind, and health. It is a condition of the whole. The joining of wellness and fitness in our life is a condition of the mind, body, and soul.

The Interchangeability of Wellness, Fitness and Health

As stated previously, being fit and being well are totally different conditions. Your wellness rating is dependent upon your immune system, and what vitamins, supplements, and nutrition you provide for your immune system. Fit people can sometimes be unwell. And well people can sometimes be unfit

Most individuals do not take the time to completely understand the health advantages of being both fit and well. We read and absorb the information we're given through the media and health organizations, without ever pondering if we're receiving all the information we need, or simply the part that is profitable to be seen or heard. Fitness gyms need your monthly fees in order to remain operational. They have no real concern about the condition of your immune system. Physical fitness is a condition of the body alone. Hospitals and doctors need you as a patient in order to remain operational; they want you to know you need to be fit and well, but often leave out important pieces that affect your wellness and, therefore, your ability to be fit.

What about eating habits? What about vitamins? What role does our daily intake play in our health, our wellness, and our fitness? More than you have been lead to believe or understand. The body's ability to remain well under anything other than ideal conditions is a

direct result of the nutrition received on a daily basis. The mind's ability to remain well is, again, a direct result of our nutrition intake. For instance, the human brain doesn't develop well without the necessary input of protein in our daily diet

You pick up the magazines each day, and you're bombarded with health and fitness information. Advertisements and articles that are designed to impart much needed information to the reader about the state of fitness and health in America today, and what we as responsible citizens should do. I want you to stop, and think for just one moment. How do you determine your current fitness and wellness levels? Does your regular doctor as you each time you go if you believe yourself to be fit and well? Probably not. Nor does he give you any method for determining the status on your own. Fitness centers abound in this country, and most are staffed with counselors who can test your fitness level. What about your wellness level? Are they one and the same? They are not one and the same, yet they rely heavily on each other to keep you healthy.

The terms are often used interchangeably. Quite often someone will talk about their health, when they're really addressing a fitness issue. Then you will encounter conversations where the word wellness is used to discuss a health issue. Because these issues are still new as far as the participating public is concerned, there will continue to be confusion as to the proper use of each term. It's not so important that we use the correct term, just that we take an active role in our wellness, fitness and overall health.

The same is true when considering our quality of life, what role does our overall health and wellness play in the quality of our life?

The Quality of Life: Is Health Important?

As a matter of course, all responsible persons should take the time to educate themselves, and their children, about the benefits of healthy eating. Learning to eat for life in a health conscious way is one of the best guarantees for a long and fulfilling life. The quality of our lives is as important as the quantity to most individuals, but because of debilitating disease, we are often forced to make a decision and choose between quality and quantity.

Thanks to the advances in modern medicine, the average person's life span now exceeds seventy years. If you stop to think, that's quite a long time to walk around on this earth. Along with the wonderful life expectancy increases, however have the detrimental effects of overeating and unhealthy eating. It seems that as we advance in one area, we regress in others

The issue of obesity brings this debate to the forefront, what kind of quality life can someone who can barely walk because of their weight have? The first question I always ask, is how did we get here? How did we go from one of the most physically fit nations, to just wallowing in our weight? I believe the answer lies in our lack of education about the weight gaining process, and a lack of concern about our children learning how to eat and exercise correctly.

Today, we must determine how much nourishment we need, how much physical exercise we need, and how best to accomplish those ends. Calorie needs, nutritional needs, physical needs, and education about those needs now is information we should all understand, at least as it applies to our individual self. If you will visit your local doctor, library, or fitness center, there is massive amounts of information available to help educate and to help you make good health choices, no matter what the age group.

The question raised in the title of this article, would have a resounding YES as the answer. The life you choose to lead, no matter what your field of interest, your level of education, or your level of income, your life is tremendously affected by your health. Maintaining your health is one of the most important things you can do as an individual to enjoy what time you have on this earth. It is also one of the most important things you can do for you family. As we become an older population, and our life expectancy increases, do we want to become burdens on our children? Or de we want our time with our children in our retirement years to be something we and they have enjoyed?

There are so many things to do in life that allow us to enjoy the fruits of our labor. All of these options can be cut short if we haven't taken the time to take care of ourselves.

Quality is as important as quantity. Education of the healthy choices we can make, making the right health choices, and then living life to the fullest should be the ultimate goal of every person alive.

Speaking of education, before we can make really effective choices, we need to have a complete comprehension of the subject at hand.

Wellness Terminology

There are many words today associated with wellness. Many of those terms are new for readers, and some of the terms are interchangeable between fitness, wellness, and health. So let's take a minute to explain some of the terms you may see from time to time.

Wellness itself is defined as the condition of good physical and mental health, especially when maintained by proper diet, exercise, and habits.

Meditation, an exercise recommended for everyone, but especially those of use with hectic, stressful lifestyles, is defined as an engagement in contemplation, especially of a spiritual or devotional nature. Meditation has been shown to be an effective method of lowering blood pressure, relieving stress, and promoting overall good health, by simply reflecting upon our day, and finding happiness within ourselves.

Fitness refers to the condition of our physical body and

mental fitness would of course be addressing our mental state. Often we will join and participate in fitness centers that provide personal trainers, and stationary fitness equipment. There are numerous pieces of equipment available that perform many different exercises to address specific areas of the body. The best time to learn about this equipment is during the orientation session of the fitness center you have chosen.

Exercise covers a lot of ground. There are so many forms of exercise that we can only try to cover some of the more popular and well defined programs. There are aerobic programs that focus on heart rate and your cardio health. There are water aerobics that again focus on your heart health. Weight training and free weights are used for building muscle mass, and sculpting the body. Walking is one of the best exercises available, as it doesn't jar our bodies, but uses all parts for toning and building heart rate. Running, swimming, jogging, and skiing are all forms of exercise, but not recommended for the novice.

Your nutritional needs refer to the physical supplements of vitamins, minerals and calories needed in order for you to sustain optimum physical health. Much discussion is centered on this topic right now, because our nation faces obesity problems of epidemic proportions.

Alternative therapies refer to the alternative medicine options such as chiropractic care, acupuncture, herbal cures, and holistic medicine. Of the examples given here, chiropractic and acupuncture are becoming more widely accepted as complements to the traditional form of western medicine. Studies are conducted often that support the evidence that chiropractic care and acupuncture are effective forms of medicine.

Herbal cleansing and healing are terms used by many of the natural healers to describe what ingestion of certain herbal combinations can provide for the body in the effort to bring it back to optimal health, or to sustain optimal health.

Today wellness is used not only in conjunction with health and fitness, but also wellness of the mind, body, and spirit.

There is an ever increasing movement among the health conscious citizens, that wellness should include not only our physical being, but our mental and spiritual health. The only true form of wellness must include the entire person.

What Makes Us Well?

Wellness refers to the condition of good physical and mental health, especially when maintained by proper diet, exercise, and habits. Nutrition refers to the nurturing of our body, in our ability to keep it healthy and functioning as it is supposed to do. Our ability to provide the body with all the necessary food, vitamins, and minerals so that we continue to thrive in our daily life processes. But what makes us well?

The first place to start would be with the examination of your eating habits. Since we are a product of what we eat, if our eating habits are unhealthy, or do not provide for the nutrition we need, we're not going to be healthy individuals at the end of the process. Do you take in more calories than your body needs? Are you supplementing your vitamins and minerals to make sure you are getting your recommended daily allowances? If you're not making the most basic of efforts to take care of your nutritional needs, you aren't a well individual.

Next, you might want to look at your exercise habits, if there are any. If there aren't any exercise routines to examine, no wellness. Everyone, no matter what their age, benefits from exercise. Whether it is organized exercise activities, free weights, or simply establishing a personal routine, exercise is an excellent wellness tool. It keeps our bodies conditioned, our mental sharpness working at top speed, and thanks to the physical aspect, we get a boost to our cardio health, extra calorie burn, and more oxygen to those cells!

Being able to deal with and handle the daily stresses of life keeps us well. Making sure we take the time to accommodate our needs for stress relief, such as downtime, therapy time, massage time, or simply take the time for a nice, hot bath. The body tends to retain stress in the muscle of the shoulder and back. Taking the time to relax, do relaxation exercises, and
combine this with physical exercise for the entire body, and you shouldn't have any trouble maintaining a state of wellness.

Our personal habits either keep us well or prevent us from being well. If you smoke, drink, or lose sleep to excess you're not the well individual you could be. Smoking, drinking, and loss of sleep work to our detriment, and it takes extreme discipline to stop. Smoking fills our body with carcinogens, and works to keep us tired and lethargic.

Giving ourselves adequate time to devote to all areas of our physical needs, from our nutritional intake needs, to our physical fitness needs, to the need for quite time contributes to our level of wellness. How well we allocate time for these needs, and the choices we make in fulfilling these needs, keeps us well.

There are so many occasions to stop and question our efforts at maintaining optimal health, that we usually don't even take the time to begin the examination. But it is beneficial to our overall health, the quality and quantity of our life, to make every effort to be well, healthy, individuals.

Wellness

You pick up the magazines each day, and you're bombarded with health and fitness information. Advertisements and articles that are designed to impart much needed information to the reader about the state of fitness and health in America today, and what we as responsible citizens should do. I want you to stop, and think for just one moment. How do you determine your current fitness and wellness levels? Does your regular doctor as you each time you go if you believe yourself to be fit and well? Probably not. Nor does he give you any method for determining the status on your own. Fitness centers abound in this country, and most are staffed with counselors who can test your fitness level. What about your wellness level? Are they one and the same? They are not one and the same, yet they rely heavily on each other to keep you healthy.

Being fit and being well are totally different conditions. Your wellness rating is dependent upon your immune system, and what vitamins, supplements, and nutrition you provide for your immune system. Fit people can sometimes be unwell. And well people can sometimes be unfit. However, when you do combine the two, and use sound principles based on clean living, exercise, and healthy eating, you attain a state of equilibrium where you are both fit and well.

Most individuals do not take the time to completely understand the advantages of being both fit and well. We read and absorb the information we're given through the media and health organizations, without ever pondering if we're receiving all the information we need, or simply the part that is profitable to be seen or heard. Fitness gyms need your monthly fees in order to remain operational. They have no real concern about the condition of your immune system. Physical fitness is a condition of the body alone. Hospitals and doctors need you as a patient in order to remain operational; they want you to know you need to be fit and well, but often leave out important pieces that affect your wellness and, therefore, your ability to be fit.

What about eating habits? What about vitamins? What role does our daily intake play in our health, our wellness, and our fitness? More than you have been lead to believe or understand. The body's ability to remain well under anything other than ideal conditions is a

direct result of the nutrition received on a daily basis. The mind's ability to remain well is, again, a direct result of our nutrition intake. For instance, the human brain doesn't develop well without the necessary input of protein in our daily diet. No protein, no intelligence. No intelligence, then none of the other states is attainable.

Our spiritual input is a determining factor when establishing our wellness level. We all need the benefit of spiritual reflection, as a way of cleansing ourselves of the toxins of our daily life. Spirituality is a way of assuring ourselves of a renewing, and rebirth of ourselves as caring humans. Wellness encompasses our state of being, mind, and health. It is a condition of the whole. Wellness is a condition of the mind, body, and soul.

Information on Wellness

What is wellness and where do we go to learn about wellness? Wellness is defined as our overall good health, and the condition sustained by healthy eating and fitness habits. We have so many places to turn for wellness information, that it would be impossible to cover all the
possibilities in one article. However, we'll cover the most common places to look, and let the reader take it from there.

The major sources of wellness information are available to everyone, everywhere. Libraries, the internet, your physical fitness instructor, and your health teachers are all viable avenues of information sources. The library contains more information about health and wellness than you could possibly read in a year's time. There are magazines, periodicals, medical journals, and all sorts of books written on ways to become fit, to maintain fitness, or to participate in fitness activities. There are sources of information that explain the benefits of being well, the physical benefits, the mental benefits, the social benefits, and the self-esteem and emotional benefits.

The library will also usually have video and audio information available on almost any topic covered by the reading material. They may even have wellness tapes available for viewing. Often, the library provides the opportunity for the low-income to access materials that otherwise would not be available. Video and audio tapes are examples of this opportunity.

The internet opens more windows on wellness than the library, since the internet is a compilation of many libraries, news articles, newspapers, and individual input. You have only to type in the word wellness using one of the available search engines, and suddenly you've got more sources of information than you can research. The search engines often return information in the order of actual relevance to your search words. So bear that in mind as you search. The first couple of pages will contain the most relevant information on wellness. You can locate information about wellness, local wellness programs, and instructors who specialize in one-on- one wellness evaluations and personal attainment plans.

Your local school physical education instructor and health teachers are invaluable sources of wellness information, in that they have an education in health and well-being. They are privy to the most sought after reliable sources of real wellness benefits. Many of the articles you will find, and much of the information you read, is not 100% accurate, ask a teacher, or instructor actually involved in wellness programs, and you are going to receive much more accurate feedback

Your federal government publishes massive quantities of information about the health and wellness in this country, from many different perspectives. The United States Department of Agriculture is responsible for determining our daily recommended allowances, and as such, accumulates much information about wellness programs, the state of physical and mental wellness in the United States, and how well we participate in wellness programs.

How Do We Evaluate Wellness?

Wellness of the body occurs when all the body processes, physical and mental are functioning as the peak levels. What does it take to achieve a complete body wellness? It requires more than simply taking a trip to the gym, or a walk in the park.

To evaluate our state of wellness, we must establish the goals we achieve through being well. We make our lives more enriched and easier to live. We are able to reap the benefits of well thought out plans of diet and exercise many years into our life, just because we have taken the time to remain well and fit.

Your immune system is a tale tell sign of your state of wellness and one of the real benefits of a healthy, well immune system is the prolonging of the onset of many age-related diseases. Conditions such as macular degeneration, Alzheimer's, strokes, heart attacks, and overall feelings of good health depend upon a healthy immune system.

Our ability to continue in a normal routine many years past the accepted age of retirement is a goal achieved through maintaining a state of wellness. To many older people, their work becomes a genuine source of enjoyment. Work no longer appears as the thief of our free time, it becomes an old friend that we are accustomed to visiting with. It can become a reason to continue to get up and go about our day. Either way, our ability to continue participating is a direct benefit of our state of wellness and continued good health.

In evaluating our wellness goals, and state of being, the mental capacity for continued learning, teaching, and experiencing is a top priority. Mental sharpness comes from continued use of the mind to learn, communicate and think. The benefit of retaining those resources is felt even longer than the benefit of physical wellness.

What about the physical benefits of continued wellness? The peace of mind that comes from knowing your body is in top shape, ready to deal whatever comes along, is a priceless possession. To be able to ascertain that you've spent your day wisely, and invested in yourself is a real accomplishment. The benefit seen from adding just 20 minutes of exercise to your daily routine are unbelievable. I can attest to the tremendous increase in energy, as a participant in walking for exercise. I lost a total of 74 lbs. in one year, by simply adding walking to may routine. I had been dieting for almost two months, with very little in the way of results. Walking was suggested by my physician, and I've never been so impressed. My energy levels were three times what they were prior to beginning the exercise program. Increased energy levels are one of the greatest benefits of a well and fit body.

Continued wellness and evaluation of our level of wellness is a lifetime responsibility.
If we use our resources wisely and educate our selves about the things our body needs to
maintain wellness, over the duration of our life, it isn't a difficult thing to attain. The benefits of continued wellness are reaped will into our later years. Look at it as an investment you make, not of dollars and cents, but of time and education. The return on your investment is as yet unmatched by any prescription available.

What Are Your Wellness Needs?

As we go about our busy lives, our wellness needs doesn't often come to mind. In fact, probably until you read the title of this article, it never even crossed your mind. But even when we are well, we have needs that help us to sustain that wellness. Have you ever given thought to what those needs are?

Your wellness rating is dependent upon your immune system, and what vitamins, supplements, and nutrition you provide for your immune system. Nutrition comes in the form of our daily intake of food our eating habits determine the value of our daily nutritional intake.

What about vitamins? What role do vitamins and minerals play in our wellness needs? More than what some of you have been lead to believe or understand. The body's ability to remain well under anything other than ideal conditions is a direct result of the nutrition received on a daily basis. The mind's ability to remain well is, again, a direct result of our nutritional intake. However, when you use sound principles based on clean living, exercise, and healthy eating, you attain a state of equilibrium where you are meeting your nutritional wellness needs

What about our preventive needs for our physical body? Alternative medicine, holistic medicine, and meditation all address different areas of preventive maintenance for our physical health.

We don't often think of the chiropractor until some part of our body isn't functioning as it should, most often our back. But what about chiropractic care for the well individual? Is it a benefit to the well person, to visit a chiropractor when really nothing is wrong? You bet it's a benefit and here's why.

The very nature of chiropractic care is the belief in the body's own healing properties.

Quite often, we can have small problems in one area of our body, and not even realize it until the effect is felt in a much larger way, somewhere else.

The practice of chiropractic care focuses on the relationship between your spine and your nervous system. The spine is the structure, and the nervous system is the function. Chiropractic believes these two systems work in unison to keep and then restore your body's health.

Acupuncture is the basic foundation for Traditional

Chinese Medicine and is based on the belief that there are two opposing and inseparable forces within our body. They are known as the Yin and Yang of the entire person. The Yin is representative of the cold, slow, or passive principle, and yang represents the hot, excited or active principle. A healthy state is achieved by maintaining a balance state of the yin and yang. This is done through vital pathways or meridians that allow for the flow of qi, or vital energy. The vital energy flow occurs along pathways known as meridians. These meridians connect over 2,000 acupuncture points along the body. There are 12 main meridians, and 8 secondary meridians. Although traditional western medicine does not completely understand how acupuncture works, the proof that it does work has been shown in several studies conducted by western medical facilities.

Meditation is the other form of preventive maintenance that we need as we maintain our overall wellness. Meditation is preventive maintenance for the mind. Meditation gives us the opportunity to reflect on our inner self. To listen to that small inner voice that is supposed to help guide and direct our mental processes, but in modern day existence, is often drowned out due to excessive noise pollution.

Wellness of the Body

Wellness refers to the condition of good physical and mental health, especially when maintained by proper diet, exercise, and habits. Nutrition refers to the nurturing of our body, in our ability to keep it healthy and functioning as it is supposed to do. Our ability to provide the body with all the necessary food, vitamins, and minerals so that we continue to thrive in our daily life processes

Wellness of the body occurs when all the body processes, physical and mental are functioning as the peak levels. What does it take to achieve a complete body wellness? It requires more than simply taking a trip to the gym, or a walk in the park.

Many factors come into play when we consider our body's wellness. The daily intake of food, vitamins, and water are absolute necessities, and most often the items thought about.

What about the conditioning of our body to deal with life each day?

Does our physical exercise have anything to do with the wellness of our body?

Absolutely. For one condition without regard to the other, is not a complete whole. The body includes all of our physical processes, our mind, and our physical being as a whole. When we give thought to the wellness of the body, most often we contemplate our physical condition as it applies to our cardiovascular needs and our weight. But our bodies are much more than heart and a nice figure. What about all of our other organs? Are they well? How do we maintain a wellness of the entirety? Daily physical exercise that benefits the body as a whole, taking time to rest and restore what has been depleted from our body over the course of the day, and making sure that we adequately supply our entire body with the nutrition necessary for healthy function.

If we use our resources wisely and educate our selves about the things our body needs to maintain wellness, over the course of our life, it isn't a difficult thing to attain. But you cannot abuse your body for years, and then hope for immediate results in trying to attain an overall wellness. It didn't become unwell overnight, and it won't become well again that quickly.

Proper attention to the physical needs of each part of your body results in the wellness of the whole. Every part of your physical body exists to work in unison with another part of the body. Two hands are necessary for optimal functioning of the limbs, two feet, two eyes, etc.

The physical body is designed to work better than any machine invented to date. It is more complex and powerful than any piece of equipment we have on the market. It takes more abuse than believable, and continues to operate, even without the daily requirements being met, for several days. It is a fascinating machine, as machines go. But it is an even more fascinating temple, when we choose to care for our bodies as the temples they really are. They house our mind and soul, and when the body is well, it does a tremendous job of providing for our needs.

Wellness of the Spirit

Wellness of the spirit refers to our ability to cope with the everyday stresses and strains of living our life. Quite often, the ability to cope overwhelms us, and if we don't give sufficient time to the wellness of the spirit, or soul, we lose our ability to function properly.

Today, the evidence of that inability exists in the form of anxiety attacks. The attacks can range from extremely mild to unbelievably severe. What is happening to us when we experience anxiety attacks? Our system goes into a form of shock. I refer to as a sort of "soul shock"; nothing is physically wrong that should cause us to become ill, and nothing is wrong mentally that should cause us to experience the panic; it is within our spirit that we have lost control.

This loss of control can be momentary, or it can last for years. The most debilitating part of the process is the inability to function even in the most usual of routines. Short trips to the grocery store become impossible, because of the panic they create within the person.

Having experienced these panic attacks for a brief period of time, I can attest to their reality. It is a frightening event that only serves to add to the panic. The person experiencing these attacks feels as if they have lost control over their ability to function. They cannot meet deadlines; they aren't able to provide for their family, there are a host of reasons that cause us to come to the place of loss of control.

I believe the hectic pace of life in this 21st century only serves to enhance the need to give our spirit, our soul, our inner voice a chance to be heard. We drown out any opportunity to connect with ourselves during the course of our day, because we schedule everything, multi-task everything, and leave no down time for a conversation with our self. It's impossible to listen to your inner needs, if you're talking on the phone, listening to the radio, or interacting with your children.

At the same time this era has taken from us any chance meeting of our spiritual needs, it has also provided more opportunity for planned downtime. We have audio, video, and even massage clinics that offer us the chance to slow down and connect with our inner self. Never before has there been so much available to help us help our selves. What is the hold up? The biggest detriment is our lack of discipline and devotion to our own health and well-being. What we tend to forget during this age of super-human feats, is that the only way to sustain the super- human person, is to keep that person, all aspects of that person, well.

Wellness comes through concentrated effort, discipline, and devotion, to our body, mind and soul. The wellness of our spirit or soul affects all other parts of our person, as evidenced in the presence of panic attacks, mental breakdowns, and the inability to cope. The need to attend to our wellness needs should be added to our daily "to do" list, so that we schedule in enough time for our selves!

Wellness of the Mind

Our spiritual input is a determining factor when establishing our wellness level. We all need the benefit of spiritual reflection, as a way of cleansing ourselves of the toxins of our daily life. Spirituality is a way of assuring ourselves of a renewing, and rebirth of ourselves as caring humans. Wellness encompasses our state of being, mind, and health. It is a condition of the whole. Wellness is a condition of the mind, body, and soul.

Meditation is preventive maintenance for the mind. Meditation gives us the opportunity to reflect on our inner self. To listen to that small inner voice that is supposed to help guide and direct our mental processes, but in modern day existence, is often drowned out due to excessive noise pollution.

Our spirituality and meditation practices are the tools we have available to keep our mind as well as we keep our bodies. The mind is a complicated and versatile machine, but it can
become overwhelmed and unable to function correctly, if we don't take the time to keep it well and cared for.

Our mind has varying levels of operation, known as brainwaves. As we pass through the different stages of our day, we enter various stages of brain wave activity. The brain uses this tool as one way to allow us time to rest our busy mind, and cope with all the pieces of information we've received, a way to kind of "mind file" for the day.

When we don't give adequate time for these processes, or we simply don't get enough rest, our mind cannot maintain its state of wellness, just like our bodies aren't capable of wellness if there is no chance to rest and replenish.

Modern alternative medicine and holistic healers believe in the power of the energy that flows through our bodies; this energy radiates from our mind as well. It is believed to be the chief from of transportation for our body nervous system to carry out communication.

Breathing techniques, music, aromas, and candle therapy are all ways we utilize the opportunities to reflect on our day, allow our mind to rest and replenish itself for further use.

We must remember over the course of our daily

routine, to make time to maintain mental wellness, as we strive to maintain physical wellness. The nice thing about the whole process is that, as we go about accomplishing these tasks, quite often the opportunities for preservation and care are interchangeable. We can help to quite our mind as we take our twenty minute walk. Or we have the opportunity to build muscle strength as we meditate.

Often just the opportunity to listen to music will allow our mind the chance it needs to relax and regroup. It's not always the most formal of occasions that we find an available chance to reflect and listen to that inner voice. It can be in the middle of the day, with the wind blowing through your hair, and the radio turned up really loud!

Benefits of Meditation for the Wellness of Ourselves

Meditation, an exercise recommended for everyone, but especially those of us with hectic, stressful lifestyles, is defined as an engagement in contemplation, especially of a spiritual or devotional nature. Meditation has been shown to relieve stress, and promote overall good health, by simply reflecting upon our day, and finding happiness within ourselves. This and other mind exercises help us to keep our mind fit, and functioning at top performance levels. But up until the last twenty years, meditation was something the western world new little about. Is it necessary for our health? Or have we just come up with a new fad, to fill up the empty hours of our day?

Our mind has varying levels of operation, known as brainwaves. As we pass through the different stages of our day, we enter various stages of brain wave activity. The brain uses this tool as one way to allow us time to rest our busy mind, and cope with all the pieces of information we've received, a way to kind of "mind file" for the day.

Modern alternative medicine and holistic healers believe in the power of the energy that flows through our bodies; this energy radiates from our mind as well. It is believed to be the chief from of transportation for our body's nervous system to carry out communication.

Breathing techniques, music, aromas, and candle therapy are all ways we utilize the opportunities to reflect on our day, allow our mind to rest and replenish itself for further use. But are these methods keeping us mentally fit? Yes, it does help to keep us mentally fit. The great benefit in meditation, however, the mind's ability to transform itself into a vehicle for higher awareness.

Meditation is a way for us to become aware of the fact that there is more to our being than just our physical activity. We have so much more potential locked away in our mind, resources that we never tap into until we have the chance to quiet the mind, quiet our surroundings and open the door to the possibilities we don't examine on a day to day basis.

In our meditative state, thoughts that never have the opportunity to be heard during the bustle of the day are afforded the opportunity to come forward and be heard. Every step that we take is a step in some direction for our life. The opportunity to set our own destiny, develop our manifestation of what we believe our life should be, is the opportunity meditation provides. Every action we've ever taken started as a thought. The thought was then brought into reality by our action on that thought. So are we able to produce new thoughts and new possibilities, in this time of quiet reflection.

It is in these small moments of creativity and higher conscious operation that our mind heals itself from the stresses of the everyday activities, and maintains a real level of healthy
operation. Our mind is like our body, we don't have to look unhealthy to be unhealthy, and sooner or later, the illnesses show.

Do We Need Meditation?

Meditation, an exercise recommended for everyone, but especially those of us with hectic, stressful lifestyles, is defined as an engagement in contemplation, especially of a spiritual or devotional nature. Meditation has been shown to relieve stress, and promote overall good health, by simply reflecting upon our day, and finding happiness within ourselves. This and other mind exercises help us to keep our mind fit, and functioning at top performance levels. But up until the last twenty years, meditation was something the western world new little about. Is it necessary for our health? Or have we just come up with a new fad, to fill up the empty hours of our day?

Well, the empty hours don't exist for most of us, and quite frankly, without the opportunity to reflect and relax, I would quite possibly go completely mad Our spirituality and meditation practices are the tools we have available to keep our mind as fit as we keep our bodies. The mind is a complicated and versatile machine, but it can become overwhelmed and unable to function correctly, if we don't take the time to keep it cared for.

Our mind has varying levels of operation, known as brainwaves. As we pass through the different stages of our day, we enter various stages of brain wave activity. The brain uses this tool as one way to allow us time to rest our busy mind, and cope with all the pieces of information we've received, a way to kind of "mind file" for the day.

Modern alternative medicine and holistic healers believe in the power of the energy that flows through our bodies; this energy radiates from our mind as well. It is believed to be the chief from of transportation for our body's nervous system to carry out communication. Breathing techniques, music, aromas, and candle therapy are all ways we utilize the opportunities to reflect on our day, allow our mind to rest and replenish itself for further use. But are these methods keeping us mentally fit? Yes, it does help to keep us mentally fit. The great benefit in meditation, however, the mind's ability to transform itself into a vehicle for higher awareness.

Meditation is a way for us to become aware of the fact that there is more to our being than just our physical activity. We have so much more potential locked away in our mind, resources that we never tap into until we have the chance to quiet the mind, quiet our surroundings and open the door to the possibilities we don't examine on a day to day basis.

In our meditative state, thoughts that never have the opportunity to be heard during the bustle of the day are afforded the opportunity to come forward and be heard. Every step that we take is a step in some direction for our life. The opportunity to set our own destiny, develop our manifestation of what we believe our life should be, is the opportunity meditation provides. Every action we've ever taken started as a thought. The thought was then brought into reality by our action on that thought. So are we able to produce new thoughts, new possibilities, in this time of quiet reflection.

Quiet Reflection: A B12 Shot for the Spirit?

Modern alternative medicine and holistic healers believe in the power of the energy that flows through our bodies; this energy radiates from our mind as well. It is believed to be the chief from of transportation for our body's nervous system to carry out communication. Breathing techniques, music, aromas, and candle therapy are all ways we utilize the opportunities to reflect on our day, allow our mind to rest and replenish itself for further use. The great

benefit in meditation, however, is the mind's ability to transform itself into a vehicle for higher awareness. Meditation is a way for us to become aware of the fact that there is more to our being than just our physical activity. We have so much more potential locked away in our mind, resources that we never tap into until we have the chance to quiet the mind, quiet our

surroundings and open the door to the possibilities we don't examine on a day to day basis. Our spirit is the real benefactor in these moments of quiet reflection and meditation.

Everyday, time after time, our spirit would soar if given the opportunity. But quite often, the opportunity is stolen thanks to the ever pressing issues of job responsibilities, children, and household responsibilities. Our spirit is generally all used up by the end of the day.

In our meditative state, thoughts that never have the opportunity to be heard during the bustle of the day are afforded the opportunity to come forward and be heard. Every step that we take is a step in some direction for our life. The opportunity to set our own destiny, develop our manifestation of what we believe our life should be, is the opportunity meditation provides. Every action we've ever taken started as a thought. The thought was then brought into reality by our action on that thought. So are we able to produce new thoughts and new possibilities, in this time of quiet reflection.

It is in these small moments of creativity and higher conscious operation that our mind heals itself from the stresses of the everyday activities, and maintains a real level of healthy operation. Our spirit has the opportunity to renew. Revive. Like the dying patient that receives the administration of CPR in the final hour, our spirit receives the moments of solitude that allow it to regroup, regain that wonderful faith in ourselves and mankind. Our mind is like our body, we don't have to look unhealthy to be unhealthy, and sooner or later, the illnesses show, unless we're given the opportunity for rebirth of our basic beliefs. This is how we provide the nourishment needed for our spirit to remain healthy.

Some people choose to accommodate this through community worship, some people through moments of quiet solitude in nature. Still others choose renewal through silent meditation and prayer. No matter our choice of activity the important accomplishment lays in the renewal of our spirituality and our belief in mankind.

Are You Well?

Wellness refers to the condition of good physical and mental health, especially when maintained by proper diet, exercise, and habits. Nutrition refers to the nurturing of our body, in our ability to keep it healthy and functioning as it is supposed to do. Our ability to provide the body with all the necessary food, vitamins, and minerals so that we continue to thrive in our daily life processes. But do we know if we are really well? How do we tell?

The first place to start would be with the examination of your eating habits. Since we are a product of what we eat, if our eating habits are unhealthy, or do not provide for the nutrition we need, we're not going to be healthy individuals at the end of the process.

Do you take in more calories than your body needs? Are you supplementing your vitamins and minerals to make sure you are getting your recommended daily allowances? If you're not making the most basic of efforts to take care of your nutritional needs, you aren't a

well individual. You may not look sick, you may not have any noticeable symptoms of ill-health, but you're not the well individual you could be.

Next, you might want to look at your exercise habits, if there are any. If there aren't any exercise routines to examine, no wellness. Everyone, no matter what their age, benefits from exercise. It keeps our bodies conditioned, our mental sharpness working at top speed, and thanks to the physical aspect, we get a boost to our cardio health, extra calorie burn, and more oxygen to those cells!

What about the stress levels in your life? Do work in an environment with high levels of stress? Is your personal life a source of comfort or does it add to your stress levels? Do you engage in some form of stress-relieving activity?

Stress is the number on contributor to heart attacks and strokes, since they manage to speed up the affect of the real culprits. Stress is basically an out of control situation for most adults today. We manage to schedule every moment of our free time, and leave ourselves with no time for quiet reflection, or time to deal with life's unexpected emergencies.

Stress brings us to the next two topics of health abuse. Smoking and drinking are often used to offset the effect that stress has on our nervous system. These solutions however do not provide any real help. If you smoke, drink, or lose sleep to excess, you're not the well individual you could be. Smoking, drinking, and loss of sleep work to our detriment, and it takes extreme discipline to stop. Smoking fills our body with carcinogens, and works to keep us tired and lethargic.

There are so many occasions to stop and question our efforts at maintaining optimal health, that we usually don't even take the time to begin the examination. But it is beneficial to our overall health, the quality and quantity of our life, to make every effort to be well, healthy, individuals.

Now, where does fitness begin to enter into the equation? Before we begin a length discussion about fitness, let's make sure we understand exactly what fitness is, and some of the terms we're going to use.

Fitness Terminology

There are many words today associated with fitness. Many of those terms are new for readers, and some of the terms are interchangeable between fitness, wellness, and health. So let's take a minute to explain some of the terms you may see from time to time.

Fitness is defined differently from different sources, but the overall meaning of fitness is our ability to function with vigor and alertness throughout the course of our day to day responsibilities.

Fitness refers to the condition of our physical body and mental fitness would of course be addressing our mental state. Often we will join and participate in fitness centers that provide personal trainers, and stationary fitness equipment. There are numerous pieces of equipment available that perform many different exercises to address specific areas of the body. The best time to learn about this equipment is during the orientation session of the fitness center you have chosen.

Meditation, an exercise recommended for everyone, but especially those of use with hectic, stressful lifestyles, is defined as an engagement in contemplation, especially of a spiritual or devotional nature. Meditation has been shown to be an effective method of lowering blood pressure, relieving stress, and promoting overall good health, by simply reflecting upon our day, and finding happiness within ourselves.

Your nutritional needs refer to the physical supplements of vitamins, minerals and calories needed in order for you to sustain optimum physical health. Much discussion is centered on this topic right now, because our nation faces obesity problems of epidemic proportions.

Alternative therapies refer to the alternative medicine options such as chiropractic care, acupuncture, herbal cures, and holistic medicine. Of the examples given here, chiropractic and acupuncture are becoming more widely accepted as complements to the traditional form of western medicine. Studies are conducted often that support the evidence that chiropractic care and acupuncture are effective forms of medicine.

Herbal cleansing and healing are terms used by many of the natural healers to describe what ingestion of certain herbal combinations can provide for the body in the effort to bring it back to optimal health, or to sustain optimal health.

Fitness

You pick up the magazines each day, and you're bombarded with health and fitness information. Advertisements and articles that are designed to impart much needed information to the reader about the state of fitness and health in America today, and what we as responsible citizens should do. I want you to stop, and think for just one moment. How do you determine your current fitness and wellness levels? Does your regular doctor ask you each time you go if you believe yourself to be fit and well? Probably not. Nor does he give you any method for determining the status on your own. Fitness centers abound in this country, and most are staffed with counselors who can test your fitness level. What about your wellness level? Are they one and the same? They are not one and the same, yet they rely heavily on each other to keep you healthy.

Being fit and being well are totally different conditions. Your wellness rating is dependent upon your immune system, and what vitamins, supplements, and nutrition you provide for your immune system. Fit people can sometimes be unwell. And well people can sometimes be unfit. However, when you do combine the two, and use sound principles based on clean living, exercise, and healthy eating, you attain a state of equilibrium where you are both fit and well.

Most individuals do not take the time to completely understand the advantages of being both fit and well. We read and absorb the information we're given through the media and health organizations, without ever pondering if we're receiving all the information we need, or simply the part that is profitable to be seen or heard. Fitness gyms need your monthly fees in order to remain operational. They have no real concern about the condition of your immune system. Physical fitness is a condition of the body alone. Hospitals and doctors need you as a patient in order to remain operational; they want you to know you need to be fit and well, but often leave out important pieces that affect your wellness and, therefore, your ability to be fit.

What about eating habits? What about vitamins? What role does our daily intake play in our health, our wellness, and our fitness? More than you have been lead to believe or understand. The body's ability to remain well under anything other than ideal conditions is a
direct result of the nutrition received on a daily basis. The

mind's ability to remain well is, again, a direct result of our nutrition intake. For instance, the human brain doesn't develop well without the necessary input of protein in our daily diet. No protein, no intelligence. No intelligence, then none of the other states is attainable.

Our spiritual input is a determining factor when establishing our fitness level. We all need the benefit of spiritual reflection, as a way of cleansing ourselves of the stress of our daily life. Spirituality is a way of assuring ourselves of a renewing, and rebirth of ourselves as humans. Fitness encompasses our body's health, as a whole and in this respect it includes the mind. It is a condition of the whole body. Fitness is a condition of wellness for our physical body.

Information on Fitness

What is fitness and where do we go to learn about fitness? Fitness is our ability to function with alertness and energy over the course of our daily activities. We have so many places to turn for fitness information, that it would be impossible to cover all the possibilities in one article. However, we'll cover the most common places to look, and let the reader take it from there.

The major sources of fitness information are available to everyone, everywhere. Libraries, the internet, your physical fitness instructor, and your health teachers are all viable avenues of information sources. The library contains more information about health and fitness than you could possibly read in a year's time. There are magazines, periodicals, medical journals, and all sorts of books written on ways to become fit, to maintain fitness, or to participate in fitness activities. There are sources of information that explain the benefits of being fit, the physical benefits, the mental benefits, the social benefits, and the self-esteem and emotional benefits. The library will also usually have video and audio information available on almost any topic covered by the reading material. They may even have fitness tapes available for viewing. Often, the library provides the opportunity for the low-income to access materials that otherwise would not be available. Video and audio tapes are examples of this opportunity.

The internet opens more windows on fitness than the library, since the internet is a compilation of many libraries, news articles, newspapers, and individual input. You have only to type in the word fitness using one of the available search engines, and suddenly you've got more sources of information than you can research. The search engines often return information in the order of actual relevance to your search words. So bear that in mind as you search. The first couple of pages will contain the most relevant information on fitness. You can locate information about fitness, local fitness center locations, and instructors who specialize in one-on-one fitness plans.

Your local school physical education instructor and

health teachers are invaluable sources of fitness information, in that they have an education in fitness. They are privy to the most sought after reliable sources of real fitness benefits. Many of the articles you will find, and much of the information you read, is not 100% accurate, ask a teacher, or instructor actually involved in the fitness process, you are going to receive much more accurate feedback

Your federal government publishes massive quantities of information about the fitness in this country, from many different perspectives. The United States Department of Agriculture is responsible for determining our daily recommended allowances, and as such, accumulates much information about fitness alternatives, the state of fitness in the United States, and how well we participate in fitness programs.

Past these sources, check out your local fitness center. Quite often they have random information posted, current magazines, and periodicals that address current fitness issues and often offer interested persons the chance to observe fitness in action

What Are Your Fitness Needs?

As we go about our busy lives, our fitness needs do not often come to mind. In fact, probably the only thought that is given to our fitness needs relates to the 15 pounds we think we need to lose. But even when we are fairly fit, we have needs that help us to sustain that fitness. Have you ever given thought to what those needs are?

Meditation, an exercise recommended for everyone, but especially those of us with hectic, stressful lifestyles, is defined as an engagement in contemplation, especially of a spiritual or devotional nature. Meditation has been shown to relieve stress, and promote overall good health, by simply reflecting upon our day, and finding happiness within ourselves.

Your nutritional needs levels are dependent upon your eating habits and whether you use daily supplements of vitamins and minerals in order for you to sustain optimum physical health. Much discussion is centered on this topic right now, because our nation faces obesity problems of epidemic proportions.

Our eating habits make up a large portion of our nutritional daily intake. What we consume goes a long way to keeping our bodies fit.

Do we understand what our nutritional requirements are, how to fulfill those requirements, and how to look for real nutritional value in our foods? I'm not sure that nutrition has been successfully addressed in its own right. We hear nutrition in relation to our vitamin intake, our fortified cereals and milk, and in the context that we need "nutritional value" from our food choices. But what really is nutrition when applied to our daily bodily functions? Nutrition refers to the nurturing of our body, in our ability to keep it healthy and functioning as it is supposed to do. Our ability to provide the body with all the necessary food, vitamins, and minerals so that we continue to thrive in our daily life processes. Quite often, our vitamin and mineral needs outweigh our caloric needs. In those instances, we turn to manufactured vitamins and minerals to fill the gap.

Alternative medicine options such as chiropractic care,

acupuncture, herbal cures, and holistic medicine are all ways we can help to keep ourselves fit. All of these alternative healing approaches offer ways to incorporate their use into staying fit and healthy. Of the examples given here, chiropractic and acupuncture are becoming more widely accepted as complements to the traditional forms of exercise and nutrition. Herbal cleansing and healing are used by many to provide for ways for body keep itself in a state of fitness and optimal health.

What role does exercise play in this process? Well, exercise conditions our body to keep it in optimal shape. To keep muscles functioning correctly and build muscle mass. The more muscle mass we have, the more calories we burn. The more calories we burn, the better our metabolism is at using up the calories we take in through food consumption. Can you begin to see how our body is really a well functioning machine? It's a continual circle of events, one feeding off the other. When all the events are coming together properly, we are healthy, happy individuals.

Today, we must determine how much nourishment we

need, how much physical exercise we need, and how best to accomplish those ends. Calorie needs, nutritional needs, physical needs, and education about those needs now is information we should all understand, at least as it applies to our ability to maintain our fitness levels. If you will visit your local doctor, library, or fitness center, there is massive amounts of information available to help educate and to help you make good health choices, no matter what the ultimate goal, fitness maintenance, or fitness improvement.

Energy Levels for the Fit

Fitness itself is defined as the ability of the human body to function with vigor and alertness, without undue fatigue and with ample energy to engage in leisure activities, and to meet physical stresses.

Fitness refers to the condition of our physical body and mental fitness would of course be addressing our mental state. When our bodies are physically fit, we should have enough energy to address all of the activities that are faced by our peers, and at the end of the day, still have some energy left for our families.

Learning to incorporate fitness into our daily routine is where the biggest obstacle to fitness is placed. Many of us would truly benefit from being more physically fit; we simply do not want to devote the time it would take to condition our bodies. We would rather sit at the table and chat with our friends or tune in to the latest hit television series, than devote thirty minutes each day to our health.

Walking is one of the most productive forms of exercise, and causes a tremendous increase in our energy levels. The benefit seen from adding just 20 minutes of walking to your daily routine are unbelievable.

I can attest to the tremendous increase in energy, as a participant in walking for exercise. I lost a total of 74 lbs. in one year, by simply adding walking to may routine. I had been dieting for almost two months, with very little in the way of results. Walking was suggested by my physician, and I've never been so impressed. My energy levels were three times what they were prior to beginning the walking, and I truly enjoyed the peace of mind that I achieved during those daily walks.

I think exercise and being fit does something for a person's self-esteem, and the mind. Deeper forms of relaxation accompany physical fitness. When meditation is incorporated into the routine, the energy levels continue to soar. When you are able to relax, and truly enjoy the way your body feels, and the accomplishment of a day's tasks, you can renew physically for the next day, overnight. That's one of the greatest benefits of exercise and fitness, tremendous energy.

Physically, what is happening to us as we become more fit? It's a process that has been addressed so many times, but we fail to make the connection most of the time. Our metabolic process is a finely tuned process. When we have it working at maximum capacity, we feel great. We're eating right, exercising, and our metabolism is making the most of those calories we're consuming. It fires up and runs, into overdrive if necessary, in order to keep that energy
coming. It's a concept our forefathers really didn't need to understand, because their living conditions kept them physically fit. Today, however we've become quite sedentary, and our
livelihood no longer requires us to physically work, we do the mental work all day, and sit while we are on the job. No physical activity interferes with our preprogrammed way of living. Our bodies still function just like our grandfather's needed. But we've changed the process, our
bodies haven't.

That's why we still need to keep physically fit, If not through our work, we need recreational routines to accomplish that task. It will keep us healthy, running at top speed, and feeling great!

Metabolism: What Is It?

The dictionary defines metabolism as the sum of all biochemical processes involved in life, or the sustaining of life. In application concerning our health, metabolism is related to the intake and use of food. In reference to the case in point it is our ability to utilize our food to the fullest extent.

Some people have really high rates of metabolism. In other words, when they consume food, their bodies burn it up almost as fast as then consume it. Then there are those of use who use our food intake so slowly, as to not even notice that we're burning calories. These people who burn quickly are often slim and trim, the people who burn more slowly are the people with a tendency toward obesity.

The body's metabolism is a unique process for each individual person. No two people metabolize food at the same rate therefore no two people have the metabolism. We all use our calories at different rates, with different results. Our metabolism, like our fingerprints is unique to each of us. But the need to understand and accommodate this metabolism is an issue that we all face.

All of this metabolic process is related to our calorie intake, our vitamin and nutrition needs, our thyroid and endocrine production, and how well all of these processes come together. For years, people have sought ways to raise the metabolic rate. If you can raise someone's metabolic rate, you are then better able to control the burn of calories, especially for overweight or obese people. This would make the goal of better or improved health a much easier reality for those people. Efforts to date have produced very little results. There are foods that we can consume that naturally raise our metabolic rate, but not to a great extent. What we need is a way to directly alter the rate. We need to be able to raise our metabolism to a point where we can actually see a benefit.

What determines our metabolic rate, as far as our genetics? Generally, we tend to inherit the same tendencies for metabolic rates, body frames, and other related body functions from our parents. Thus, the origin of "well, she comes from big people; naturally she's going to be big".

Right now, the greatest results in raising our metabolism come from exercise and building our muscle mass, while reducing our body fat. Adding more muscle to the body, in turn causes us to burn more calories, and this helps to elevate our metabolic rate.

Our metabolism functions also depend on how well we have taken care of our nutritional needs. The process of burning calories and creating energy is a delicate one, and one which must be carefully tended, or it can become imbalanced. It is often through these natural imbalances that we tend to "inherit' our metabolic rate.

I believe through careful analysis, and attention to each person's unique needs, we could bring about a more natural balance of the metabolic burn vs. the calorie intake. To a level where optimal health and weight control are in equilibrium.

Metabolism for the Fit Individual

The dictionary defines metabolism as the sum of all biochemical processes involved in life, or the sustaining of life. In application concerning our health, metabolism is related to the intake and use of food. In reference to the case in point it is our ability to utilize our food to the fullest extent.

Right now, the greatest results in raising our metabolism come from exercise and building our muscle mass, while reducing our body fat. Adding more muscle to the body, in turn causes us to burn more calories, and this helps to elevate our metabolic rate.

Our metabolism functions also depend on how well we have taken care of our nutritional needs. Some people have really high rates of metabolism. In other words, when they consume food, their bodies burn it up almost as fast as then consume it. Then there are those of use who use our food intake so slowly, as to not even notice that we're burning calories. These people who burn quickly are often slim and trim, the people who burn more slowly are the people with a tendency toward obesity.

The body's metabolism is a unique process for each individual person. No two people metabolize food at the same rate therefore no two people have the metabolism. We all use our calories at different rates, with different results. Our metabolism, like our fingerprints is unique to each of us. But the need to understand and accommodate this metabolism is an issue that we all face.

All of this metabolic process is related to our calorie intake, our vitamin and nutrition needs, our thyroid and endocrine production, and how well all of these processes come together. For years, people have sought ways to raise the metabolic rate. If you can raise someone's metabolic rate, you are then better able to control the burn of calories, especially for overweight or obese people. This would make the goal of better or improved health a much easier reality for those people. Efforts to date have produced very little results. There are foods that we can consume that naturally raise our metabolic rate, but not to a great extent. What we need is a way to directly alter the rate. We need to be able to raise our metabolism to a point where we can actually see a benefit.

This is where the effort to stay physically fit and active provides tremendous payoff. Over the course of your life, if you stay active, exercise, and maintain optimal health for your muscles, you will see a tremendous difference in the rate that your body metabolizes food. As people age, their metabolism quite naturally slows down. The greatest way to prevent this from happening is through exercise and staying fit.

I believe through careful analysis, exercise, and attention to each person's unique needs, we could bring about a more natural balance of the metabolic burn vs. the calorie intake. To a level where optimal health and weight control are in equilibrium.

Metabolism: Can We Control It?

The body's metabolism is a unique process for each individual person. No two people metabolize food at the same rate therefore no two people have the metabolism. We all use our calories at different rates, with different results. Our metabolism, like our fingerprints is unique to each of us. But the need to understand and accommodate this metabolism is an issue that we all face.

The dictionary defines metabolism as the sum of all biochemical processes involved in life, or the sustaining of life. In application concerning our health, metabolism is related to the intake and use of food. In reference to the case in point it is our ability to utilize our food to the fullest extent.

Right now, the greatest results in raising our metabolism come from exercise and building our muscle mass, while reducing our body fat. Adding more muscle to the body, in turn causes us to burn more calories, and this helps to elevate our metabolic rate.

Our metabolism functions also depend on how well we have taken care of our nutritional needs. Some people have really high rates of metabolism. In other words, when they consume food, their bodies burn it up almost as fast as then consume it. Then there are those of use who use our food intake so slowly, as to not even notice that we're burning calories. These people who burn quickly are often slim and trim, the people who burn more slowly are the people with a tendency toward obesity.

For years, people have sought ways to raise the metabolic rate. If you can raise someone's metabolic rate, you are then better able to control the burn of calories, especially for overweight or obese people. This would make the goal of better or improved health a much easier reality for those people. Efforts to date have produced very little results. There are foods that we can consume that naturally raise our metabolic rate, but not to a great extent. What we need is a way to directly alter the rate. We need to be able to raise our metabolism to a point where we can actually see a benefit.

This is where the effort to stay physically fit and active provides tremendous payoff. Over the course of your life, if you stay active, exercise, and maintain optimal health for your muscles, you will see a tremendous difference in the rate that your body metabolizes food. As people age, their metabolism quite naturally slows down. The greatest way to prevent this from happening is through exercise and staying fit.

The best way to date to control our metabolic process is through proper nutrition, daily exercise, eating the foods known to have an effect on our metabolic rate, and plenty of rest. The metabolic process can be indirectly controlled by the methods we just discussed. Direct control is not available, to date.

I believe through careful analysis, exercise, and attention to each person's unique needs, we could bring about a more natural balance of the metabolic burn vs. the calorie intake. To a level where optimal health and weight control are in equilibrium.

Obesity in Adolescents

You see it everyday, news and information that bring
to the front our problem with our weight. It is a national
problem. It's not just your older sedentary population; it's
not just your overworked middle-age population; and it's not
just your nerdy teenage population. It is a national epidemic.

The first question I always have, is how did we get
here? How did we go from one of the most physically fit
nations, to just wallowing in our weight?

Over the last thirty years, food nutritionists and the
food industry as a whole have embraced the idea of lowering
our fat intake. This was a direct result of the information
published by the government that encouraged less egg
consumption because of the cholesterol found in eggs. After
that particular piece of information, doctors began to
discover that when we consume fat, we have higher
incidences of cholesterol problems. The logical conclusion:
fat must be bad for you. And so, an entire generation as
grown up with fat-free foods. A whole generation grew up
believing that fat was what made us fat, clogged our arteries,
and generally caused ill-health.

So what did we do? We turned to carbs to make up for the loss in taste of food that had the fat removed; for you see, fat is what gives many of our foods their delicious taste. When you remove the fat, the taste must be artificially injected into the food. The end result is a food that is higher in carbohydrate content, but lower in fat. Hence, all the wonderful labels displaying the claim of "fat free" but neglect to mention the higher level of carbohydrates. Lowered fat should have created a population of slim, trim, healthy people. Right?

We could not have been further from the truth. As it turns out, fat is a necessary part of our metabolic processes. We need the fat in order to properly utilize many of the vitamins and nutrients we consume. When did we make this discovery? Probably some thirty years too late for some people.

Now, we have an entire generation of young people, who have because of their high carbohydrate food choices, become a nation of obese adults. Never before has a nation recorded the kind of obesity problems this nation is facing now. Never before have we ever had so much, to have so little. These young people are experiencing low self-esteem, weight related health problems, and whole host of emotional problems, thanks to obesity issue. How can we try to help them correct this problem?

According to the guides published by the USDA, calorie needs vary from one age group to another, one gender to another. So how do you determine what your individual needs are? You can setup a journal for recording your daily caloric intake for about a month. Make a note of your weight each day. If you don't gain any weight during the course of that month, you're eating your recommended calorie level in order to maintain your weight. Now, take that calorie information, use the food pyramid and comprise a combination of foods that will help you achieve this recommended daily intake, and still be enough to be filling and please the palette.

You now have an individualized healthy eating plan. This is the safe sure way to reach weight loss goals. It didn't become a problem overnight, and it won't go away overnight.

Fitness of the Body

Bodily fitness is being able to deal with and handle the daily stresses of life, good physical and mental health, especially when maintained by proper diet, exercise, and habits. Nutrition refers to the nurturing of our body, in our ability to keep it healthy and functioning as it is supposed to do. Our ability to provide the body with all the necessary food, vitamins, and minerals so that we continue to thrive in our daily life processes is a part of overall fitness.
Fitness refers to the condition of good physical, mental, and spiritual health.

Fitness of the body occurs when all the body processes, physical and mental are functioning as the peak levels. What does it take to achieve complete body fitness? It requires more than simply taking a trip to the gym, or a walk in the park.

Many factors come into play when we consider our body's fitness. The daily intake of food, vitamins, and water are absolute necessities, and most often the items thought about. What about the conditioning of our body to deal with life each day?

Does our physical exercise have anything to do with

the fitness of our body? Absolutely. For one condition without regard to the other, is not a complete whole. The body includes all of our physical processes, our mind, and our physical being as a whole. When we give thought to the fitness of the body, most often we contemplate our physical condition as it applies to our cardiovascular needs and our weight. But our bodies are much more than heart and a nice figure. What about all of our other organs? Are they fit? How do we maintain a fitness of the entirety? Daily physical exercise that benefits the body as a whole, taking time to rest and restore what has been depleted from our body over the course of the day, and making sure that we adequately supply our entire body with the nutrition necessary for healthy function.

If we use our resources wisely and educate our selves about the things our body needs to maintain fitness, over the course of our life, it isn't a difficult thing to attain. But you cannot abuse your body for years, and then hope for immediate results in trying to attain overall fitness. It didn't become unfit overnight, and it won't become fit again that quickly.

Proper attention to the physical needs of each part of

your body results in the fitness of the whole. Every part of your physical body exists to work in unison with another part of the body. Two hands are necessary for optimal functioning of the limbs, two feet, two eyes, etc.

The physical body is designed to work better than any machine invented to date. It is more complex and powerful than any piece of equipment we have on the market. It takes more abuse than believable, and continues to operate, even without the daily requirements being met, for several days. It is a fascinating machine, as machines go. But it is an even more fascinating subject, when we choose to care for our bodies as the temples they really are. They house our mind and soul, and when the body is fit, it does its job tremendously well.

Fitness of the Spirit

Fitness of the spirit refers to our ability to cope with the everyday stresses and strains of living our life. Quite often, the ability to cope overwhelms us, and if we don't give sufficient time to the fitness of the spirit, or soul, we lose our ability to function properly.

Today, the evidence of that inability exists in the form of anxiety attacks. The attacks can range from extremely mild to unbelievably severe. What is happening to us when we experience anxiety attacks? Our system goes into a form of shock. I refer to as a sort of "soul shock"; nothing is physically wrong that should cause us to become ill, and nothing is wrong mentally that should cause us to experience the panic; it is within our spirit that we have lost control.

This loss of control can be momentary, or it can last for years. The most debilitating part of the process is the inability to function even in the most usual of routines. Short trips to the grocery store become impossible, because of the panic they create within the person.

Having experienced these panic attacks for a brief period of time, I can attest to their reality. It is a frightening event that only serves to add to the panic. The person experiencing these attacks feels as if they have lost control over their ability to function. They cannot meet deadlines; they aren't able to provide for their family, there are a host of reasons that cause us to come to the place of loss of control.

I believe the hectic pace of life in this 21st century only serves to enhance the need to give our spirit, our soul, our inner voice a chance to be heard. We drown out any opportunity to connect with ourselves during the course of our day, because we schedule everything, multi-task everything, and leave no down time for a conversation with our self. It's impossible to listen to your inner needs, if you're talking on the phone, listening to the radio, or interacting with your children.

At the same time this era has taken from us any chance meeting of our spiritual needs, it has also provided more opportunity for planned downtime. We have audio, video, and even massage clinics that offer us the chance to slow down and connect with our inner self. Never before has there been so much available to help us help our selves. What is the hold up? The biggest detriment is our lack of discipline and devotion to our own health and well-being. What we tend to forget during this age of super-human feats, is that the only way to sustain the super- human person, is to keep that person, all aspects of that person, well.

Fitness comes through concentrated effort, discipline, and devotion, to our body, mind and soul. The fitness of our spirit or soul affects all other parts of our person, as evidenced in the presence of panic attacks, mental breakdowns, and the inability to cope. The need to attend to our fitness needs should be added to our daily "to do" list, so that we schedule in enough time for our selves!

Fitness of the Mind

Meditation, an exercise recommended for everyone, but especially those of us with hectic, stressful lifestyles, is defined as an engagement in contemplation, especially of a spiritual or devotional nature. Meditation has been shown to relieve stress, and promote overall good health, by simply reflecting upon our day, and finding happiness within ourselves. This and other mind exercises help us to keep our mind fit, and functioning at top performance levels

Our spirituality and meditation practices are the tools we have available to keep our mind as fit as we keep our bodies. The mind is a complicated and versatile machine, but it can become overwhelmed and unable to function correctly, if we don't take the time to keep it cared for.

Our mind has varying levels of operation, known as brainwaves. As we pass through the different stages of our day, we enter various stages of brain wave activity. The brain uses this tool as one way to allow us time to rest our busy mind, and cope with all the pieces of information we've received, a way to kind of "mind file" for the day.

When we don't give adequate time for these processes, or we simply don't get enough rest, our mind cannot maintain its state of fitness, just like our bodies aren't capable of fitness if there is no chance to rest and replenish.

Modern alternative medicine and holistic healers believe in the power of the energy that flows through our bodies; this energy radiates from our mind as well. It is believed to be the chief from of transportation for our body's nervous system to carry out communication.

Breathing techniques, music, aromas, and candle therapy are all ways we utilize the opportunities to reflect on our day, allow our mind to rest and replenish itself for further use. But are these methods keeping us mentally fit? Yes, but they don't work alone. The absorption of new information, new opportunities to learn, and creative play provide our mind the stimulus it needs in order to stay fit and functioning.

The onset of many age-related mental disorders occurs because we haven't taken the time to keep our mind youthful, and involved in new learning. Learning new things forces our mind to form new neural pathways. We need those neural pathways for the transmission of information from the body to the mind, or with our ability to form new memories. If we don't exercise the mind, we lose the fitness.

We must remember over the course of our daily routine, to make time to maintain mental fitness, as we strive to maintain physical fitness. The nice thing about the whole process is that, as we go about accomplishing these tasks, quite often the opportunities for preservation and care are interchangeable. We can help to quite our mind as we take our twenty minute walk. Or we have the opportunity to build muscle strength as we meditate.

Often just the opportunity to listen to music will allow our mind the chance it needs to relax and regroup. It's not always the most formal of occasions that we find an available chance to reflect and listen to that inner voice. It can be in the middle of the day, with the wind blowing through your hair, and the radio turned up really loud!

Are You Fit?

Fitness refers to ability of the body to function with vigor and alertness. Nutrition refers to the nurturing of our body, in our ability to keep it healthy and functioning as it is supposed to do. Our ability to provide the body with all the necessary food, vitamins, and minerals so that we continue to thrive in our daily life processes. But do we know if we are really fit? How do we tell?

First, you might want to look at your exercise habits, if there are any. If there aren't any exercise routines to examine, no fitness. Everyone, no matter what their age, benefits from exercise. It keeps our bodies conditioned, our mental sharpness working at top speed, and thanks to the physical aspect, we get a boost to our cardio health, extra calorie burn, and more oxygen to those cells!

Do you take in more calories than your body needs? Are you supplementing your vitamins and minerals to make sure you are getting your recommended daily allowances? If you're not making the most basic of efforts to take care of your nutritional needs, you aren't a fit individual. You may not look sick, you may not have any noticeable symptoms of ill-health, but you're not the fit and toned individual you could be.

What about the stress levels in your life? Do work in an environment with high levels of stress? Is your personal life a source of comfort or does it add to your stress levels? Do you engage in some form of stress-relieving activity?

Stress is the number on contributor to heart attacks and strokes, since they manage to speed up the affect of the real culprits. Stress is basically an out of control situation for most adults today. We manage to schedule every moment of our free time, and leave ourselves with no time for quiet reflection, or time to deal with life's unexpected emergencies.

Fitness requires us to examine more than just our exercise routine. The mere definition of fitness refers to the body's ability to meet physical stresses. That includes coping with our day to day life, getting from the beginning of the day to the end, without being worn completely out. In order to be truly fit, we find ways to rid ourselves of built up stress, the kind that begins to affect our muscles, muscle tone, and composition. Massages are the best cure for ridding our bodies of the stress buildup that can occur, even with exercise regimens and detract from our overall fitness.

Exercises that demand total body involvement are the best for maintaining and improving your level of fitness most effectively. Running, swimming, jogging, dancing, cycling, and very brisk walking are some of the more popular total body involvement exercises.

There are so many occasions to stop and question our efforts at maintaining optimal health, that we usually don't even take the time to begin the examination. But it is beneficial to our overall health, the quality and quantity of our life, to make every effort to be fit, healthy, individuals.

Where You Live Affects Your Fitness

During the course of your growing up years, you lived wherever your parents chose to live. You didn't give any thought to the health implications of the location your parents chose, or if they had chosen a place that was conducive to your physical, mental, and spiritual health.

Chances are your parents didn't give it much thought either. Not until recently, has there ever been given any thought to the fact that where you live affects your level of fitness. But it does, and it's a piece of information that is sure to influence many generations to come.

So how is this information compiled, and what can we learn from it? The information is compiled based on statistical information from areas such as smog levels, pollution levels, water quality, government based fitness incentives, and recreational and fitness facilities available. Generally, one of the major magazines published in the United States, will compile all this statistical data, and publish an article as a recreational guide to healthy cities.

What do we learn from all this published information? That where we live really does affect our health and well-being, and sometimes, there's very little we can do about changing that fact. Unless, of course, you want to move.

Often, the greatest contributor to our health and fitness, via our outside environment, is the level of pollution we're forced to live with on a daily basis. How do we absorb pollutants in our outside environment? The most common way is through the air we breathe. It is not the only way, however. The water we drink, the homes we live in, and the cars we drive, all have the potential for unhealthy contaminants.

Our work environment at one time was a contributor to the pollutants we were exposed to, but thanks to greater Environmental Protection regulation, most of those dangers have been eradicated.

Past the pollutants contribution, the availability of health facilities, the amount of government support for health and fitness, and the availability of medical faculties also affects our health and wellness from a location standpoint. If you live in a rural area with no direct access to health facilities, and there is no medical facility, your level of fitness and health will not compare to that of a person who lives in a more populated area that can offer those things. The down side to the more populated area, of course, is a greater risk of air pollution.

Some areas of this country are just fitness conducive. Places where the air is still free from pollutants, there is an availability of hiking, biking, and walking trails, and the medical and fitness facilities are numerous. The problem with most of those places, however is that they are mostly of a recreational base, not manufacturing or otherwise industrialized, and jobs are not that numerous.

What can you do about your own fitness concerns, based on where you live? Make the most of where you are. Educate yourself about the greatest fitness problems in your area, and do what you can to make corrections for your own fitness benefit.

Fitness Centers: An Investigation

Today, we have many Americans who are obsessed with health, and yet we are a nation of obese individuals. Obesity in this country has reached epidemic proportions, and we have more available than at any other time in history to help us control our weight. What is the problem? Why do we still have health issues, when we have some many health facilities available?

There are facilities that cater to the young, the old, the male, the female. There are 24 hour facilities, facilities that offer daycare, individualized programs, youth programs, organized classes, and fitness assessments.

It would seem with all these choices, that Americans would not have any problem controlling their weight, their health or their overall wellness. Many fitness centers offer the new client an opportunity for an initial assessment, personalized training plans, and continued consultation services, free with their membership.

If you happen to be a mother, with small children, many of the fitness facilities offer built in daycare facilities. You are free to exercise, while your children play in a supervised and safe setting. If you also happen to feel uncomfortable exercising in mixed company, there are fitness centers that offer men only or women only exercise times. If not designated times, often they have segregated facilities.

What about Pilates, aerobics and other forms of organized and instructed toning and cardiovascular health? Most fitness facilities have that covered also. Upon joining a gym or center you are usually provided a schedule of classes that are being taught, and the times that they are taught. Then once each month, you will receive a newsletter and calendar that provides updated information about facility changes, class offerings and any other points of interest.

There is just simply no reason that a person could not locate a fitness that suits his or her needs and become a part of the health movement. Cost is usually not an issue, either. Today, many companies offer free memberships for their employees in an effort to cut medical expense and lost time due to sickness and injuries. On the average, a healthy employee costs an employer $1000 dollars less each year, than the coworker who does not participate in health and fitness programs. That simply takes medical costs into consideration. What about lost productivity due to illness or injury?

If you find that your company doesn't offer such a plan, the monthly expenditure for a membership to the gym, should more than pay for itself in the course of your attaining a level of increased health. You should see a decrease in your medical bills, and over the counter health needs, simply because your body is in a better position to fight off germs and bacteria.

Fitness centers and gyms across this country open each day, to provide persons form all walks of life, a better chance at health; to afford each person the opportunity to work toward overall wellness and a fit and conditioned body.

It is up to each individual to take advantage of that opportunity.

Does Your Income Affect Your Health?

Our level of income directly affects our health. Did you know that? How much money you make helps to determine how healthy you will be. Doesn't really make sense, if you don't' look at the broader picture. In the big picture, however, here is the view: you are educated, have a degree, and are exposed to tons of information during your college years. You are exposed to health classes, athletes, and all sorts of professional people who already understand the importance of health in your life.

You graduate college, your income levels are quite nice, and you have the opportunity to purchase magazines, health and fitness of course. Can you see how your education and intelligence levels affect your health now? This is a generalization that has proven itself time and again. All you have to do is observe your developed countries versus the third world, underdeveloped countries. Standard of living and health are directly related. Past the consideration of intelligence development, our level of education and income plays a tremendous role in our ability to educate ourselves about the health options we should exercise. Affordable fitness centers are one of the nicer privileges of higher income. Most fitness centers provide their customers with individualized weight and exercise programs that further advance the

customer's health.

Having higher income levels provides us with access to fitness centers, better choices for our eating patterns, and better medical care.

It is in the final section of the previous sentence that there is found a real benefit of higher income, in direct relation to our health. Higher levels of education and income almost always have access to better medical care. The availability of better care, whether it is through better company paid insurance, life in a metropolitan area versus rural area, or simply being able to afford a more specialized doctor when the situation warrants.

In most cases, higher income families live in more

populated areas, with access to better doctors and larger medical facilities. Often their employers have nurses or doctors that are retained, if not on staff, as emergencies warrant.

If the evidence presented above is not enough to satisfy your curiosity concerning the role income plays in our health, take the time to visit the US Census. This information is available through the internet. There you will find all kinds of statistics, from income averages in areas of the United States, to education levels in those same places. Also available is information related to the household. Check for yourself. You can see a direct relationship in many areas of the country between income levels and health statistics for that area.

It is sad indeed, that many of the people who are in the greatest need are not able to get that need met. Socialized medicine as been studied as a possible solution to our some of our health problems, but when studied in detail, socialized medicine really does not improve the level of health for the population, it just makes medical care free and generally of less quality.

What Role Does Our Intelligence Play in Our Health?

This is a double sided coin. Does health affect intelligence? Yes. Does intelligence affect health? Yes. This is one of those wonderful situations where the cause and effect works both ways. What happens in one area, will generally affect the other.

It is a known and proven fact, that the eating and health habits we use as children, directly affects our level of development. This includes the brain. Protein, one of the most
important basic life building blocks, works directly in the brain's development. No protein, no proper development.

Well, it doesn't take very much intuition here, to notice if the brain doesn't develop to optimal operation levels, you will not have a health conscious individual. Generally, you do not have individuals develop to become productive, prosperous citizens, and certainly not healthy, productive, prosperous citizens.

Past the consideration of intelligence development, our level of education and intelligence plays a tremendous role in our ability to educate ourselves about the health options we should exercise. With generations prior to the 20th century, physical energy expenditures used up whatever nutritional resources you had provided earlier. Physical work and a real lack of nutritional supplements kept the body in constant need of nourishment. That is a time past.

Today, with the advent of the computer, physical activity is no longer a part of the work equation. We no longer lack for vitamins and minerals, thanks to the boom in the vitamin market.

Today, we must determine how much nourishment we need, how much physical exercise we need, and how best to accomplish those ends. Calorie needs, nutritional needs, physical needs, and education about those needs now is information we should all understand, at least as it applies to our individual self.

Our level of income directly affects our health. Did you know that? How much money you make helps to determine how healthy you will be. Doesn't really make sense, if you don't' look at the broader picture. In the big picture, however, here is the view: you are educated, have a degree, and are exposed to tons of information during your college years. You are exposed to health classes, athletes, and all sorts of professional people who already understand the importance of health in your life.

You graduate college, your income levels are quite nice, and you have the opportunity to purchase magazines, health and fitness of course. Can you see how your education and intelligence levels affect your health now? This is a generalization that has proven itself time and again. All you have to do is observe your developed countries versus the third world, underdeveloped countries. Standard of living and health are directly related.

If the evidence presented above is not enough to satisfy your curiosity concerning the role intelligence plays in our health, take the time to visit the US Census. This information is available through the internet. There you will find all kinds of statistics, from income averages in areas of the United States, to education levels in those same places. Also available is information related to the household. Check for yourself. You can see a direct relationship in many areas of the country between income levels and health statistics for that area.

What Role Does Nutrition Play in Our Health?

Nutrition as it applies to our daily lives means that we take in what we need to maintain our body's healthy state. Nutrition has become an important word thanks to the involvement of the USDA in our daily food requirements, and the FDA's involvement in determining what is and is not dangerous for us to consume.

What about eating habits? What about vitamins? What role does our daily intake play in our health? More than you have been lead to believe or understand. The body's ability to remain well under anything other than ideal conditions is a direct result of the nutrition received on a daily basis. The mind's ability to remain well is, again, a direct result of our nutritional

intake. For instance, the human brain doesn't develop well without the necessary input of protein in our daily diet. No protein, no intelligence.

Nutrition refers to the nurturing of our body, in our ability to keep it healthy and functioning as it is supposed to do. Our ability to provide the body with all the necessary food, vitamins, and minerals so that we continue to thrive in our daily life processes.

How do we determine that we are providing the essential nutritional needs? That knowledge comes by educating ourselves about what our individual needs are, the needs of our family, and then taking that knowledge and applying it to the foods we buy, that we prepare, and that our families consume.

Health is taught as a science course, and addresses matters of personal hygiene, diseases, and the broad spectrum of health as it applies to the masses. No individual attention is given to how to attain optimal health via our eating habits. It's funny that we skip the most important, fundamental building block to good health: our nutritional and caloric consumption in our food. I personally believe we should have the field of nutrition and physical activity married into something combined to provide every person that enters the school system with a personal knowledge of their bodies' needs, caloric, and nutritional, so that they complete their education with mental and physical competencies, as well as analytical and mathematical competence.

Nutrition is a concept that should be as important to

our educational process as our ability to count. The ability to recognize our nutritional requirements, find the foods we need to fulfill those requirements, and differentiate between healthy food consumption and "unhealthy" eating habits is not an option. Not for a healthy, happy, long, and quality life

What we should absorb as we travel along life's daily path is a way to incorporate good nutrition into our lifestyle. There is generally just as much room for good as there is bad, it just so happens that bad nutritional habits hold more appeal.

Bad nutrition receives more advertising dollars than healthy nutritional options, and is often more visible. But that doesn't mean it's any easier, more convenient, or cheaper. Habits, generally take about two weeks to make the switch from conscious action to unconscious thought. Two weeks is not long, it's not long at all for decisions that will affect you for the rest of your life. It's also not long for the potential reward that comes from setting an example your children can follow, and you can be proud for them to follow. You teach them daily about the good habits you want them to develop, and then you demonstrate a bad one in your nutrition choices. C'mon, mom and dad, let's practice what we preach.

Is There Health Without Water?

Water makes up 98% percent of our body, and without this life-giving fluid, you and I would not survive. The human body can survive for up to 3 weeks on water alone. Try surviving without the water and you might make it 4 to 5 days. It's a truly amazing and health sustaining fluid, and it's just water!

What really do we get from water, that our body must have, and can't live without? It's the benefit of the fluidity of water, and what it does for our bodies that is the most important part. All of our bodily functions rely on the cells in our bloodstream to supply them the nutrients and minerals that they need to carry out those vital functions. How do our cells achieve that end? They absorb the vitamins, minerals, and nutrients we take in during our digestive process. But they also absorb water, or liquid fluids that are a product in direct water intake or the digestive process, but either way, water must be a part of the formula. Since cells are also made of mostly water or fluid, it's necessary to keep lots of water coming, and make sure that we include at least 64 ounces in our daily intake.

Ask any health and fitness instructor, and they will tell you that you must consume plenty of water during your exercise routine, weight lifting, and physical activity requires us to take in water or some sort of sports drink. Most of the instructors will recommend just plain water.

Why must we keep our bodies so hydrated? In order for the metabolic and muscle burn to

occur, there must be plenty of water and plenty of oxygen. Oh, wait a minute, there's another benefit of water. It contains oxygen, a substance our body cannot get enough of. Water also helps to flush the lactose acid that accumulates in our muscles when we work out, or use the excessively. The lactose acid can build up and cause soreness, stiffness, and muscle pain.

So, if you look at the benefits that water supplies, and you are trying to maintain health and fitness, you can not ignore the fact that water needs to be a part of your daily intake. But how much water do we need to adequately supply our bodies, and help fuel our metabolic processes?

The most often recommended quantity is 8 eight ounce glasses each day.

Personally, I believe that amount should be closer to 10 eight ounce glasses each day.

What other benefits can water provide, other than the obvious ones of adding fluid to our bodies? Water helps keep our skin healthy and glowing. It helps in the reduction of wrinkling, and aids in our ability to flush fat, toxins, and any other unwanted or foreign substance from our bodies. Flushing our intestines with plenty of water allows us to maintain stable and safe quantities of yeast and bacteria. Plenty of water keeps our thought processes and brain function at optimal levels, and prevents headaches that are caused from not enough hydration.

It's pretty amazing what that one little glass of water can do!

Vitamins: To Be or Not to Be?

Nutrition as it applies to our daily lives means that we take in what we need to maintain our body's healthy state. Nutrition has become an important word thanks to the involvement of the USDA in our daily food requirements, and the FDA's involvement in determining what is and is not dangerous for us to consume.

But what is our responsibility in the nutrition game? Do we understand what our nutritional requirements are, how to fulfill those requirements, and how to look for real

nutritional value in our foods? I'm not sure that nutrition has been successfully addressed in its own right. We hear nutrition in relation to our vitamin intake, our fortified cereals and milk, and in the context that we need "nutritional value" from our food choices. But we don't often stop to think, what do we really need in nutritional supplements?

Vitamins and minerals are more readily available to us than ever before, and we're still no better equipped to actually determine what we need to take, than we were forty years ago. Just because we see the latest advertisement about a particular vitamin and decide the symptoms of deficiency apply to us, does not mean we need to rush out and purchase the product. The symptoms of deficiency for lots of vitamins and minerals are the same or overlapping. What we need is a way to detect, on an individual basis, what our body's lack, and then plan a suggested nutritional solution.

The complete lack of unity between our medical field and the herbal field, (this is the field that vitamins and minerals belong to) is a disgrace in a country so forward thinking as the United States. But it is also where we fall short in providing our citizenry with the tools they need to make better, informed decisions. The medical field has long resented any contact that patients might make with herbalists, vitamins and minerals, or any other proposed health aid, that wasn't directly related to medicine.

Thanks to this prevalent attitude among most all doctors, we have missed great opportunities to advance a generation's health. If you were to take a cross section of the population, and check for adequate levels of the most used and fortified vitamins and minerals, you would probably find the as high as 80% or the population is lacking in a least one of the vitamins and minerals. Now, that doesn't sound too bad, until you stop to think, what if it's calcium? A calcium deficiency brings on osteoporosis, a deteriorating of the bone. This disease alone costs millions in medical expense to the population.

Can you see how a little more cooperation and open-minded participation on the part of our medical field could result in far fewer health problems? It would also have provided the general population with a viable way to discern their vitamin and mineral needs, accurately.

Blood tests, urine tests, and other simple office procedures would provide the vast majority of the information needed for us to arm ourselves, and head off to the health store. Preventive medicine comes in all shapes, forms, and tablets!

How the Brain Affects Our Health

Almost everyone is aware today, of the importance of protein in our diet. Protein directly affects our muscles, tissues and organs. It also directly effects the development of these organs, our brain included. What happens if we don't get the necessary protein or any of the other many nutrients our body, not just our brain, needs to function correctly? It is through the use of our mind (or brain, whichever term you prefer) that we are able to absorb the necessary facts and figures and process it into useable pieces of information.

Nutrition refers to the nurturing of our body, in our ability to keep it healthy and functioning as it is supposed to do. Our ability to provide the body with all the necessary food, vitamins, and minerals so that we continue to thrive in our daily life processes.

How do we determine that we are providing the essential nutritional needs? That knowledge comes by educating ourselves about what our individual needs are, the needs of our family, and then taking that knowledge and applying it to the foods we buy, that we prepare, and that our families consume. Once again, through the use of our minds, we are able to take the guidance provided by the USDA, develop a journal and establish what our daily requirements are, so that take care of our necessary nutritional needs.

According to the guides published by the USDA, calorie needs vary from one age group to another, one gender to another. So how do you determine what your individual needs are? You can setup a journal for recording your daily caloric intake for about a month. Make a note of your weight each day. If you don't gain any weight during the course of that month, you're eating your recommended calorie level in order to maintain your weight. Now, take that

115

calorie information, check with a nutritionist about the recommended daily allowances of vitamins and minerals that you need. Take both pieces of information, calorie intake and nutritional requirements, use the food pyramid and comprise a combination of foods that will help you achieve these recommended daily intakes, and still be enjoyable food. You now have an individualized healthy eating plan.

Over the course of absorbing the instructions for a healthy, well-balanced eating plan, we have used our mind through the whole process. Our ability to think and reason, our level of education, and the exposure we receive to outside input on a daily basis affects our entire environment, but especially our health. We make choices based on the information we have previously absorbed. Our food, exercise, and recreation choices are no exception. It just so happens that these choices can immediately affect our health.

Maybe now you have a clearer picture of the opportunities we have for our brain to affect our health. It is more than just conscious decisions. It is a result of brain development through childhood, adolescence, and adulthood. It is a result information we have previously absorbed, and input we will continue to receive.

What Are Your Nutritional Needs?

Nutrition as it applies to our daily lives means that we take in what we need to maintain our body's healthy state. Nutrition has become an important word thanks to the involvement of the USDA in our daily food requirements, and the FDA's involvement in determining what is and is not dangerous for us to consume.

But what is our responsibility in the nutrition game? Do we understand what our nutritional requirements are, how to fulfill those requirements, and how to look for real nutritional value in our foods? I'm not sure that nutrition has been successfully addressed in its own right. We hear nutrition in relation to our vitamin intake, our fortified cereals and milk, and in the context that we need "nutritional value" from our food choices. But what really is nutrition when applied to our daily bodily functions?

Today, we must determine how much nourishment we need, how much physical exercise we need, and how best to accomplish those ends. Calorie needs, nutritional needs, physical needs, and education about those needs now is information we should all understand, at least as it applies to our individual self. If you will visit your local doctor, library, or fitness center, there is massive amounts of information available to help educate and to help you make good health choices, no matter what the age group.

Nutrition refers to the nurturing of our body, in our ability to keep it healthy and functioning as it is supposed to do. Our ability to provide the body with all the necessary food, vitamins, and minerals so that we continue to thrive in our daily life processes.

How do we determine that we are providing the essential nutritional needs? That knowledge comes by educating ourselves about what our individual needs are, the needs of our family, and then taking that knowledge and applying it to the foods we buy, that we prepare, and that our families consume.

Quite often, our vitamin and mineral needs outweigh our caloric needs. In those instances, we turn to manufactured vitamins and minerals to fill the gap. This is a part of our nutritional needs, also.

Nutrition is one of the most complex areas to gain useful knowledge about, because there are so many components, and because each person has their own individual needs.

Women needs differ from those of men, and older women's needs differ from those of a young girl. As we age, our needs constantly change; therefore continual education about nutrition is a fact of life.

The nutritional needs of a cardiac patient are different than those of a healthy, middle- aged hiker. Can you see the complexity of the situation now? What we really need is to develop a scale that determines the nutritional needs of our bodies on a cellular level, so that as we age, as our physical condition changes, or our health changes, we can recalculate our needs, based on cellular changes and content in our body. Individuality is the key to understanding each person's nutritional needs, and then working to educate ourselves is the key to fulfilling those nutritional needs. Good nutrition should be the ultimate goal of every person alive.

Exercise and Play: What Do We Learn?

Quite often, when our children return from afternoon play, they look exhausted, and ready for a nap. That is the most accurate description, and quite the truth. Play is hard work. It is exhausting to the mind and body of the young person, and plays an extremely important role in helping them to become productive, healthy citizens.

The role of exercise and play in a young child's life provides them with many benefits. Exercise of the body is an important part of keeping the young body fit as it grows into an adult body. When we reach adulthood, if we have had the benefit of exercise and play, we tend to continue that habit into our adult years.

What else is to be gained from the opportunities that play affords? We often participate in organized sports, coordinated play times, and are a member of a large group during all of these activities. Play on this level teaches us how to interact with our peers, develop camaraderie and perform as a team with other players. These skills are absolute necessities in today's business world. But what else is happening here, during this time of play and exercise?

What we learn in body language, coping skills, and the interaction of the mind and body during our interaction with others, is invaluable. When we learn these skills well, we not only learn how to interact with others, we learn how to interact with our self. Interact with our self? That seems like a pointless exercise, but it is an all important part of maintaining our health and wellness. There are times that our bodies try to tell us things about our physical or mental condition, and we simply refuse to listen. If we have learned how to listen to others around us when they attempt to point out a need or desire, we have a useful tool in listening to ourselves. This often can mean the difference between optimal health, and creating an unhealthy situation.

What else do we learn? We learn what our physical and mental limitations are. During play, you see children and young adolescents push themselves to the very limit. But as children, we are better able to distinguish between a real limit versus what society deems our limits. As a child, or young adult, the pressures of the world do not weigh on us as they do when we are adults. We are better keepers of the temple at ten, than we are at twenty. We are still very in tune to what our body tells us, because it is our true master as a child. As an adult, we have let outside influences master our body and mind, and dominate our time.

As you can see, the benefits to be gained during our exercise and play time as children, is a benefit to us for the remainder of our lives. Too often, we adults forget the importance of exercise and play and the principles that are to be learned from time spent in these activities. We want to rush our children into their daily responsibilities, forgetting that their chief responsibility during the younger years is the play and interaction of young minds.

The Benefits of Walking

Walking is one of the most productive forms of exercise, and causes a tremendous increase in our energy levels. The benefit seen from adding just 20 minutes of walking to your daily routine are unbelievable. I can attest to the tremendous increase in energy, as a participant in walking for exercise. I lost a total of 74 lbs. in one year, by simply adding walking to may routine. I had been dieting for almost two months, with very little in the way of results. Walking was suggested by my physician, and I've never been so impressed. My energy levels were three times what they were prior to beginning the walking, and I truly enjoyed the peace of mind that I achieved during those daily walks.

The added exertion of physical exercise is often the catalyst our bodies needed to boost weight loss into high gear. For the individual trying to loose weight, the benefits of walking far exceed an infringement on personal time, or detraction from television time that occurs. Not only is it good for your body, when you're trying to cut back, it gives you something constructive to do with your time.

Exercise also decreases our hunger pangs, increases our fluid intake, and helps our blood to circulate much better.

If there are any down-side effects to walking, it is the added pressure we put on our knees, ankles, and feet. If you already have a joint condition, such as arthritis, you might want to start very slowly, and add mileage only as you see that your body can handle what you are presently doing. Taking the time to buy good, supportive shoes, and wear leg bracing if needed can eliminate any further injury or harm. Talk to your doctor is you think you might have any of these conditions, and make sure that you are taking care of your body as you exercise it.

There are some excellent magazines and journals out there that provide a novice walker with all kinds of helpful advice and tips. Tips that offer assistance in what type of walking shoe you need, to what kind of walking sticks are best. There are many opportunities for you to participate in community events, national events, and even marathons, if you choose. From shoes to clothing tips, these magazines were a real inspiration for me, also. There are real life stories that you feel as though you could have written, that sing the praises of walking as a way of life.

The peace of mind that comes from taking a few minutes to stop and enjoy the sunset as you walk cannot be compared. Walking gives you the time we no longer take for private reflection. To ask yourself if you spent your day wisely, did you omit something that needed to be done, did you listen to your spouse when he needed to talk?

Twenty minutes out of your day to walk, contribute to your health, clear your mind, and get a glimpse of the most beautiful sunset, how can you not take advantage of an offer like that?

The Mind, Body and Soul Interconnectivity

The practice of chiropractic care focuses on the relationship between your spine and your nervous system. The spine is the structure, and the nervous system is the function. Chiropractic believes these two systems work in unison to keep and then restore your body's health. The word "chiropractic" is taken from Greek, and means "done by hand". This is exactly how chiropractic care works. The chiropractor uses his or her hands to manipulate your body, and help it to heal itself. It is the branch of the health sciences which focuses on the neuromusculoskeletal system. That's a very big word to simply say how your spine and nervous system work together. The spine is the highway for your central nervous system; if the highway is blocked or traffic is jammed, they are usually able healers. Many cultures, the Egyptians, the Greeks, the Chinese, and even the Africans have used some form of chiropractic care for hundreds of years.

Modern alternative medicine and holistic healers believe in the power of the energy that flows through our bodies; this energy radiates from our mind as well. It is believed to be the chief from of transportation for our body's nervous system to carry out communication.

Acupuncture is one of the key components of Traditional Chinese Medicine (TCM), and operates on the premise that the body is divided into two opposing and inseparable forces, the yin and yang. Yin represents the cold, slow, or passive principle, and yang represents the hot, excited or active principle. According to TCM health is achieved by maintaining a balance state of the yin and yang. This is done through the vital pathways or meridians that allow for the flow of qi, or vital energy. The vital energy flow occurs along pathways known as meridians. These meridians connect over 2,000 acupuncture points along the body. There are 12 main meridians, and 8 secondary meridians. Although traditional western medicine does not completely understand how acupuncture works, the proof that it does work has been shown in several studies conducted by western medical facilities

Finally, in the last few years, traditional western medicine has come to accept the role that your mind, body and soul have in keeping each other healthy, during daily processes, or recovering from surgery. Almost every form of healing accepts and incorporates the fact that our bodies have a "vital energy force" that flows through, from top to bottom. This "life force" as some refer to the energy, helps to keep us connected, mind, body, and soul. To come to the understanding, as modern medicine finally has, that there are certain aspects of our health that we cannot place neatly in a physical process, has been a difficult revelation for believers of the purely scientific approaches to healing and medicine.

It's impossible to separate the mind from the body, or the body from the soul. Their interconnectivity is the basis for our life's meaning and existence. It is because of this connection, that we are able to heal ourselves in the beginning.

Chiropractic Care: A Benefit to the Well Individual?

We don't often think of the chiropractor until some part of our body isn't functioning as it should, most often our back. But what about chiropractic care for the well individual? Is it a

benefit to the well person, to visit a chiropractor when really nothing is wrong? You bet it's a benefit and here's why.

The very nature of chiropractic care is the belief in the body's own healing properties.

Quite often, we can have small problems in one area of our body, and not even realize it until the effect is felt in a much larger way, somewhere else.

The practice of chiropractic care focuses on the relationship between your spine and your nervous system. The spine is the structure, and the nervous system is the function. Chiropractic believes these two systems work in unison to keep and then restore your body's health. The

word "chiropractic" is taken from Greek, and means "done by hand". This is exactly how chiropractic care works. The chiropractor uses his or her hands to manipulate your body, and help it to heal itself. It is the branch of the health sciences which focuses on the neuromusculoskeletal system. That's a very big word to simply say how your spine and nervous system work together. The spine is the highway for your central nervous system; if the highway is blocked or traffic is jammed, they are usually able healers. Many cultures, the Egyptians, the Greeks, the Chinese, and even the Africans have used some form of chiropractic care for hundreds of years.

Why has it taken so long for chiropractic care to receive its proper recognition in western medicine? Because by its very nature, it creates a divide between traditional, western philosophies and practices and what the chiropractor practices. In modern, western medicine, prescription drugs play a huge role in our healing process. To circumvent all those years of development, and investment on the part of the drug companies, is like climbing a rock cliff. It has taken many years, much evidence, and the demand of the general public to finally make progress towards the implementation chiropractic medicine as a realistic form of healing.

Chiropractic care in the western civilizations however has experienced many hurdles on its way to becoming one of best forms of back care and preventive medicine available today. To date, much research has been done and much material published on the benefits and cost- effective nature of chiropractic treatment. The number of Americans who seek chiropractic care has more than tripled in the last ten years, and continues to grow each year. It is a known fact, if you've ever visited the chiropractor, the philosophy works, your body feels better, it heals

better, and you aren't cut, drugged, and off from work for 6 weeks to recuperate. It is interesting to note here, that chiropractors are still classified as holistic healers. In other words, they believe in the whole body approach to healing. So do the acupuncturists, and the herbal healers. It would seem to me, that traditional medicine as had a lot of catching up to do, and they thought they were in the lead!

Acupuncture: A Benefit to the Well Individual?

Before we begin a discussion about the benefits of acupuncture, let's talk about the origins of acupuncture. It was first used in China over 2000 years ago, and is one of the oldest medical procedures in the world. It is a family of procedures that stimulates the anatomy of the body and helps to balance the energy flow throughout the body. It is this kind of acupuncture that is practiced in the United Sates today, through the use of tiny, metallic needles placed in affected areas and manipulated by hand or by electrical stimulation.

Acupuncture is the basic foundation for Traditional Chinese Medicine and is based on the belief that there are two opposing and inseparable forces within our body. They are known as the Yin and Yang of the entire person. The Yin is representative of the cold, slow, or passive principle, and yang represents the hot, excited or active principle. A healthy state is achieved by maintaining a balance state of the yin and yang. This is done through vital pathways or meridians that allow for the flow of qi, or vital energy. The vital energy flow occurs along pathways known as meridians. These meridians connect over 2,000 acupuncture points along the body. There are 12 main meridians, and 8 secondary meridians. Although traditional western medicine does not completely understand how acupuncture works, the proof that it does work has been shown in several studies conducted by western medical facilities.

Now, let's move to the question of does it work? According to the National Institute of Health, the answer would be yes. Acupuncture has been shown to be effective in many areas of health care. Areas such as postoperative nausea, chemotherapy side effects, osteoarthritis, low- back pain, headache, menstrual cramps, addiction, carpal tunnel syndrome, and asthma, just to name a few. The study revealed that acupuncture was able to provide pain relief, improve function and mobility of joints due to arthritis inflammation, and served to complement standard care.

Although there are many who would doubt the effectiveness of acupuncture, once they are a patient, they are believers. It has been proposed that acupuncture works and produces its effects through regulating the nervous system. The theory proposes that since acupuncture produces its effect through regulation of the nervous system, it induces the release of endorphins and immune system cells at specific sites on the body. There is also the theory that acupuncture alters the brain chemistry by the changing the neurotransmitters in the brain.

Without doubt acupuncture was a benefit in the study, and as a patient myself, I can vouch for the wonderful effect it has had on my back. Although acupuncture is classified as an alternative medicine therapy, and there is still much to be understood about the way it works, it is a proven aid in maintaining optimal health.

But what about the well individual, can acupuncture provide a benefit to them? Absolutely. Because acupuncture works off the belief that we must maintain balance of our vital energy flow in order to remain healthy, acupuncture serves as the tool for realignment. Our vital energy flow can be out of balance, and we still feel and appear quite healthy. It is in this capacity that acupuncture serves as a sort of preventive medicine. Checking and balancing the flow of energy on the meridian points in your body is like your car receiving a tune-up before it is in need of a repair.

The Benefits of Being Well

Wellness of the body occurs when all the body processes, physical and mental are functioning as the peak levels. What does it take to achieve a complete body wellness? It requires more than simply taking a trip to the gym, or a walk in the park.

The many benefits of being well make our lives more enriched and easier to live. We are able to reap the benefits of well thought out plans of diet and exercise many years into our life, just because we have taken the time to remain well and fit.

Your wellness is dependent upon your immune system, and one of the real benefits of a healthy, well immune system is the prolonging of the onset of many age-related diseases. Conditions such as macular degeneration, Alzheimer's, strokes, heart attacks, and overall feelings of good health depend upon a healthy immune system.

Our ability to continue in a normal routine many years past the accepted age of retirement is a benefit of keeping ourselves well. To many older people, their work becomes a genuine source of enjoyment. Work no longer appears as the thief of our free time, it becomes an old friend that we are accustomed to visiting with. It can become a reason to continue to get up and go about our day. Either way, our ability to continue participating is a direct benefit of our state of wellness and continued good health.

The mental capacity for continued learning, teaching, and experiencing is a direct result of our efforts to keep our selves mentally well, and fit for the opportunities and activities that present themselves over the course of our life. Mental sharpness comes from continued use of the mind to learn, communicate and think. The benefit of retaining those resources is felt even longer than the benefit of physical wellness.

What about the physical benefits of continued wellness? The peace of mind that comes from knowing your body is in top shape, ready to deal whatever comes along, is a priceless possession. To be able to ascertain that you've spent your day wisely, and invested in yourself is a real accomplishment. The benefit seen from adding just 20 minutes of exercise to your daily routine are unbelievable. I can attest to the tremendous increase in energy, as a participant in walking for exercise. I lost a total of 74 lbs. in one year, by simply adding walking to may routine. I had been dieting for almost two months, with very little in the way of results. Walking was suggested by my physician, and I've never been so impressed. My energy levels were three times what they were prior to beginning the exercise program. Increased energy levels are one of the greatest benefits of a well and fit body.

If we use our resources wisely and educate our selves about the things our body needs to maintain wellness, over the course of our life, it isn't a difficult thing to attain. The benefits of continued wellness are reaped will into our later years. Look at it as an investment you make, not of dollars and cents, but of time and education. The return on your investment is as yet unmatched by any prescription available.

Where You Live Affects Your Wellness

During the course of your growing up years, you lived wherever your parents chose to live. You didn't give any thought to the health implications of the location your parents chose, or if they had chosen a place that was conducive to your overall wellness. Chances are your parents didn't give it much thought either. Not until recently, has there ever been given any thought to the fact that where you live affects your health and wellness. But it does, and it's a piece of information that is sure to influence many generations to come.

So how is this information compiled, and what can we learn from it? The information is compiled based on statistical information from areas such as smog levels, pollution levels, water quality, government based fitness incentives, and recreational and fitness facilities available. Generally, one of the major magazines published in the United States, will compile all this statistical data, and publish an article as a recreational guide to healthy cities.

What do we learn from all this published

information? That where we live really does affect our health and well-being, and sometimes, there's very little we can do about changing that fact. Unless, of course, you want to move.

Often, the greatest contributor to our health and wellness, via our outside environment, is the level of pollution we're forced to live with on a daily basis. How do we absorb pollutants in our outside environment? The most common way is through the air we breathe. It is not the only way, however. The water we drink, the homes we live in, and the cars we drive, all have the potential for unhealthy contaminants.

Our work environment at one time was a contributor to the pollutants we were exposed to, but thanks to greater Environmental Protection regulation, most of those dangers have been eradicated.

Past the pollutants contribution, the availability of health facilities, the amount of government support for health and fitness, and the availability of medical faculties also affects our health and wellness from a location standpoint. If you live in a rural area with no direct access to health facilities, and there is no medical facility, your level of overall health will not compare to that of a person who lives in a more populated area that can offer those things. The down side to the more populated area, of course, is a greater risk of air pollution.

Some areas of this country are just fitness conducive. Places where the air is still free from pollutants, there is an availability of hiking, biking, and walking trails, and the medical and fitness facilities are numerous. The problem with most of those places, however is that they are usually recreational based, not manufacturing or otherwise industrialized, and jobs are not that numerous.

What can you do about your own fitness concerns, in relation to where you live? Make the most of where you are. Educate yourself about the greatest fitness problems in your area, and do what you can to make corrections for your own fitness benefit.

The Benefits of Being Fit

Being able to deal with and handle the daily stresses of life is a benefit afforded to the fit person. Making sure we take the time to accommodate our needs for stress relief, such as downtime, therapy time, massage time, or simply take the time for a nice, hot bath. The body tends to retain stress in the muscles of the shoulder and back. Taking the time to relax, do relaxation exercises, and combine this with physical exercise for the entire body benefits the fit and unfit.

The added exertion of physical exercise is often the catalyst our bodies needed to boost weight loss into high gear. For the individual trying to loose weight, the benefits of being fit far exceed an infringement on personal time, or detraction from television time that occurs. Not only is it good for your body, when you're trying to cut back, it gives you something constructive to do with your time. Exercise also decreases our hunger pangs, increases our fluid intake, and helps our blood to circulate much better.

The peace of mind that comes from knowing your body is

in top shape, ready to deal whatever comes along, is a priceless possession. To be able to ascertain that you've spent your day wisely, and invested in yourself is a real accomplishment. The benefit seen from adding just 20 minutes of exercise to your daily routine are unbelievable. I can attest to the tremendous increase in energy, as a participant in walking for exercise. I lost a total of 74 lbs. in one year, by simply adding walking to may routine. I had been dieting for almost two months, with very little in the way of results. Walking was suggested by my physician, and I've never been so impressed. My energy levels were three times what they were prior to beginning the exercise program. Increased energy levels are one of the greatest benefits of a fit body.

Raised self-esteem and confidence in your appearance are also benefits to keeping a fit body. A fit and healthy individual shines in how they look, how they treat others, and the pleasure they take in going about their daily activities.

How about the benefits of a fit mind? The onset of many age-related mental disorders occurs because we haven't taken the time to keep our mind youthful, and involved in new learning. Learning new things forces our mind to form new neural pathways. We need those neural pathways for the transmission of information from the body to the mind, or with our

ability to form new memories. If we don't exercise the mind, we lose the fitness. There's also the added benefit of being able to participate as a productive citizen, well into our retirement years. For many older citizens, keeping their bodies and minds fit means that they are also able to continue to interact in their chosen work profession, keeping them continually active, and serving as a continued source of enjoyment.

Music: Our Connection to the Higher Conscious

Today, more and more seniors are watching their diet and implementing exercise programs in an effort to remain more healthful, manage stress, and participate in a lifestyle that is rewarding and enjoyable. Many are aware of the benefits of diet and exercise in helping to keep our bodies and minds operating a peak levels of performance, but what is not known is the role music can play in helping older citizens (and I believe younger ones, too) to manage stress, become a part of an enjoyable learning experience, and acquire a new tool in their efforts to stay healthy.

What many people don't realize is the role music could play in their life, throughout the course of their life. Music is our connection between the everyday spoken word, and the power of our spirituality. Music operates on sound waves that fall in the range between vocal sounds, or our voice, and spiritual prayer, or meditative brain wave lengths. What does all that say? It is a link, an avenue to connect with our higher conscious on a moment to moment basis, to relive stress, comfort us, or simply lift our spirit.

Professors and other leaders of the education

environment have long known the benefits of musical talent. Learning to make music and play musical instruments increases our mathematical and scientific analysis abilities. In the course of the learning process, the musical notations and reading of musical notes, works within the vastness of our brain to stimulate the processes associated with working mathematical problems, solving analytical problems, and excelling in the sciences.

What have we learned from watching our young people, as they learn to perform and play musical instruments? There is a direct association with the hopeful mindset of youth, and the pouring out of musical creation. Both the young mind and the musical note bring about joy and hope, in an untainted, unlearned environment. The young mind is oblivious to the constraints of life that the middle-aged person has learned well, and the musical note serves as a constant invitation to belief in the impossible.

What have studies revealed about the power of music? In studies performed on older citizens, the effect of learning to play music, and participate in music performances, lowered stress and anxiety levels, feelings of isolation and loneliness decreased, and here's the real surprise, participants actually showed increases in the production of the human growth hormone. The human growth hormone positively affects aging phenomena such as energy levels, wrinkling, osteoporosis, sexual function, muscle mass and general aches and pains.

What important information does this impart to health practitioners? It brings to the forefront the need for increased exposure to group activity and social interaction. The benefit of learning musical instruments and enjoyment of the music they generate only sees its true potential when applied in a group setting, where laughter, music and fellowship can take place. Studies of this nature serve to reinforce the long-held belief that music is a way to connect with our higher selves, our peers, and to bring about increased enjoyment of our lives.

The Yin and Yang of the Healthy Individual

The Chinese believe our bodies are complete halves, one side being the passive and the other being the aggressive, and it only through the successful union of the halves, that we have the healthy whole.

Western medicine has so far, not subscribed to this theory, in whole. There is compelling evidence to support many of the Chinese theories on the joining of the body's energy forces and balancing our flow of energy through the entire body.

Chiropractic and acupuncture philosophies base their entire practice on the successful correlation of the body's energy flow, nervous system impulses, and skeletal alignment.

What we do know, about individuals is that the entire system must be in balance for attainment of true wellness and health; our physical, mental, and spiritual existence must be aligned and working as a whole. To better understand this principle, we need to take a closer look at some of the ancient healing techniques and philosophies. Perhaps then we can develop a better understanding of how our body works with itself to heal.

In the tradition of acupuncture, the vital energy flow occurs along pathways known as meridians. These meridians connect over 2,000 acupuncture points along the body. There are 12 main meridians, and 8 secondary meridians. Although traditional western medicine does not completely understand how acupuncture works, the proof that it does work has been shown in several studies conducted by western medical facilities.

The very nature of chiropractic care is the belief in the body's own healing properties.
Quite often, we can have small problems in one area of our body, and not even realize it until the effect is felt in a much larger way, somewhere else.
The practice of chiropractic care focuses on the relationship between your spine and your nervous system. The spine is the structure, and the nervous system is the function. Chiropractic believes these two systems work in unison to keep and then restore your body's health. The word "chiropractic" is taken from Greek, and means "done by

hand".

If you take the basic premise from each form of healing, and apply it to the knowledge that we have about the interaction of the mind, body, and spirit, you can see that these ancient healing philosophies are very accurate in their belief about treatment and how the body works. They were able to discern this hundreds of years before science could actually provide the proof.

The amazing part thing to me is that with all of this knowledge, and all the opportunity for self-help and healing that we have available, we still have individuals who suffer simply
because they aren't willing to put forth the effort to learn and participate. We have every possible venue for healing options available, for the low-income, for the middle-income, and for the wealthy. There is no bias when it comes to availability. We simply need to take advantage of the yin and yang of our opportunity. Part of the halves is in place, now we just need the participants.

Right Hand vs. Left Hand: Who's Healthier?

Now, here's a tricky question. Do you suppose your health is related to your natural handedness tendencies? This is a question that has actually been studied and reviewed by member of the medical field, and to the best of their ability, there is no conclusive evidence that your natural handedness tendencies has anything to do with your state of health, or your disposition to any particular state of health.

Our overall state of health is dependent upon several factors: our diet, our exercise, our work habits, and our genetics. The first three contributors cross all natural tendency of handedness lines, and we find we have all forms of handedness in all sort of occupations, with all sorts of eating habits, and exercise habits. When you talk about our genetic disposition, you really have to understand that as a person, we received input from two parents: a mother and a father. While it is true that we normally take many of our traits from our parents, our natural tendency for handedness can come from as far back as a great-grandparent.

Our health is the culmination of inherited possibilities, and daily consistencies. We might inherit the potential for heart disease, but if we live a life of good eating habits, good exercise habits, and attend to nutritional and rest requirements; we can often overcome the inherited potential. We can glean some information from what has been learned about natural handedness tendencies to make some assumptions about a person's personality traits that might contribute to the overall health of the individual, but nothing that can be tied directly to the "handedness" of the individual.

First of all, there is only about 10% of the population that is left-handed. Now, if you're trying to conduct research, on any topic, you need a more even distribution of subject matter. If 90% of our population is right-handed, there is no way to get a proper perspective on comparative features.

The explanations of right-handed versus left-handed are still very vague generalizations, and no one group has been able to successfully explain why we are one way or the other. Since we aren't even able to agree on the reasons for the existence of a preference, how could we possibly study the health of one group versus the other, and come up with any usable information?

What we can determine are some general characteristics of one versus the other, and draw "generalizations" from that information. Most often, left-handed people are less cautious than right-handed counterparts, leading us to assume that there are more health-risks for the less cautious. Second, there is the belief that left-handed people are more creative, more extroverted than right-handers; this would lead us to assume that again, left-handed people are more exposed to opportunities for ill-health or accidents.

In all of this generalization however, there is this fact: there are more left-handed women than men, and women tend to live longer than men. This evidence simply throws all other generalizations into a quandary. Does our handedness affect our health, I think not.

Is Your Mind Playing Tricks?

Over the course of our life, our senses and our environment come together to enrich our mind, and to sometimes overwhelm our mind. Much of the knowledge we acquire comes to us through our senses. As children, we use the senses daily to absorb as much as possible. The mind is a voraciously hungry, empty den when we are young.

As we age, we depend greatly upon our senses to inform us about the world around us; hot, cold, sweet, sour, bitter, loud, soft, so many of our perceptions and actions begin with input from our five senses. There is another sense that isn't given much attention, thanks to the fact that it is centered within our body, not on the outside. But, if used properly, provides us with as much valuable information as the sense of smell, taste, touch, sight, and hearing.

Our intuition is our sixth sense. It refers to the ability to tune into the unseen world of sensing. All the other senses require a physical origin of input; our intuition does not. It requires not physical presence of an object in order for us to obtain information about the object. Thanks to the fact that we live in a materialistic world, and that most of our knowledge is dominated by the western traditions and beliefs, our ability to use our intuition is a lost art.

The eastern cultures have long used the sense of intuition and the flow of the body's natural energies to utilize the intuitive information available. The western civilizations are slow to realize the role our intuition can play in our overall health, just because it is not a "seen" source of input.

Often, our mind can seemingly play tricks on our sensory perceptions, when we fail to utilize all aspects of the six senses, we often miss some piece of the puzzle, and what seems to be complete and correct, if often lacking.

There are at times physical conditions that cause our senses to operate incorrectly, and we don't process the information correctly. This happens when we are functioning at less than optimum levels. Often this occurs during times of sickness, extreme fatigue, or due to a lack of sleep. It is at this point, that we believe our mind to play tricks on us. We believe we are receiving certain input, and in all actuality, we are not.

This is why keeping our bodies well, fit, and healthy keeps us in a reception mode to accurately process input from the outside world. It is through this accurate perception of intake that we are able to deal effectively with the world around us. All this culminates to come to this statement: in order to keep ourselves healthy and well, we must be able to accurately process
input from the world around us. It is when we lose perspective, and don't accurately "see" things as they really are that we are more likely to experience feelings of ill-

health, mental unrest, and this can lead to actually becoming ill.

Our overall wellness depends upon our ability to not only cope with our selves, but to perceive reality as it really is.

Hopefully, at the end of this report, you've gained some knowledge about the world of health, wellness, and fitness. Also, we hope you will put into practice some of the suggestions made here, in order to improve upon your life.

There are many reasons to simply read and ignore the information contained in all the individual articles, but there's one especially important reason to read, review, and put into practice everything we've talked about, for happiness, health and wellness: you.